T0271554

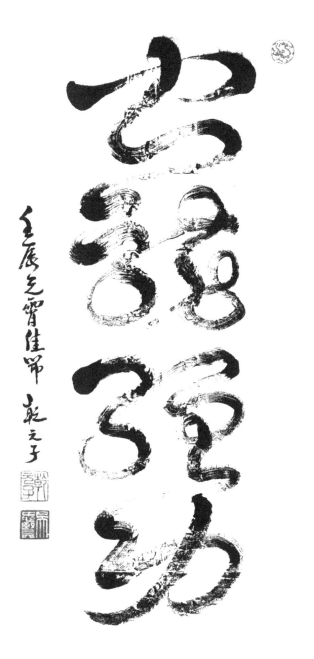

Fire Dragon Meridian Qigong

by the same author

Chinese Shamanic Cosmic Orbit Qigong
Esoteric Talismans, Mantras, and Mudras in Healing and Inner Cultivation
Master Zhongxian Wu
ISBN 978 1 84819 056 6
eISBN 978 0 85701 059 9

The 12 Chinese Animals
Create Harmony in your Daily Life through Ancient Chinese Wisdom
Master Zhongxian Wu
ISBN 978 1 84819 031 3
eISBN 978 0 85701 015 5

Seeking the Spirit of The Book of Change
8 Days to Mastering a Shamanic Yijing (I Ching) Prediction System
Master Zhongxian Wu
Foreword by Daniel Reid
ISBN 978 1 84819 020 7
eISBN 978 0 85701 007 0

Vital Breath of the Dao
Chinese Shamanic Tiger Qigong—Laohu Gong
Master Zhongxian Wu
ISBN 978 1 84819 000 9

of related interest

Chinese Medical Qigong
Editor in Chief: Tianjun Liu, O.M.D.
Foreword by Marc Micozzi, M.D., Ph.D.
Associate Editor in Chief: Kevin W. Chen, Ph.D.
ISBN 978 1 84819 023 8
eISBN 978 0 85701 017 9

FIRE DRAGON

MERIDIAN QIGONG

Essential NeiGong for Health
and Spiritual Transformation

MASTER ZHONGXIAN WU
DR. KARIN TAYLOR WU

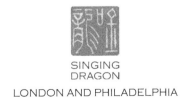

SINGING
DRAGON
LONDON AND PHILADELPHIA

First published in 2012
by Singing Dragon
an imprint of Jessica Kingsley Publishers
116 Pentonville Road
London N1 9JB, UK
and
400 Market Street, Suite 400
Philadelphia, PA 19106, USA

www.singingdragon.com

Copyright © Master Zhongxian Wu and Dr. Karin Taylor Wu 2012

All rights reserved. No part of this publication may be reproduced in any material form (including photocopying or storing it in any medium by electronic means and whether or not transiently or incidentally to some other use of this publication) without the written permission of the copyright owner except in accordance with the provisions of the Copyright, Designs and Patents Act 1988 or under the terms of a licence issued by the Copyright Licensing Agency Ltd, Saffron House, 6–10 Kirby Street, London EC1N 8TS. Applications for the copyright owner's written permission to reproduce any part of this publication should be addressed to the publisher.

Warning: The doing of an unauthorized act in relation to a copyright work may result in both a civil claim for damages and criminal prosecution.

Library of Congress Cataloging in Publication Data
A CIP catalog record for this book is available from the Library of Congress

British Library Cataloguing in Publication Data
A CIP catalogue record for this book is available from the British Library

ISBN 978 1 84819 103 7
eISBN 978 0 85701 085 8

Printed and bound in Great Britain

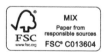

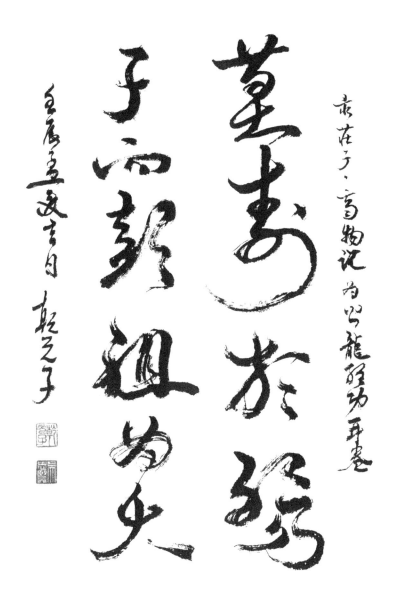

MoShouYuShangZi, ErPengZuWeiYao.

莫寿于殇子, 而彭祖为夭

There is no life longer than that of a child who has died in
infancy, while the 800-year-old sage, PengZu 彭祖 died young.

For
our son
TaiLiao Taylor Wu
吳泰了

His short journey
to this world,
his joy,
and
lovely smile
inspired us
to share the
great transformation of
Fire Dragon
with you

Contents

WORDLESS TEACHING

ChuWuWeiZhiShi, XingBuYanZhiJiao
處無為之事, 行不言之教

Attend to the action-less affairs,
Transmit the wordless teaching

LAOZI, DAODEJING

People often ask me why my masters decided to pass the secrets of their traditions on to me. Although I never asked them, I believe it was in part because I honored the traditional ways. Whenever I approached a new master to help me study Chinese medicine, martial arts, Qigong 氣功, Taiji 太極, philosophy, or Qin 琴 music, I always followed each master's guidance exactly. For at least the first few years of my training with a new master, I would never ask "Why?" Having been born and raised in a village rooted in values, customs, and a simple lifestyle not commonly found in today's world, I naturally understood the old Chinese tradition—learning comes through precise modeling of the master and from dedicating a lot of time to practice every day. Following the traditional way, I would bring questions to my masters only once I had cultivated a deep personal understanding of his or her art. Had I approached my training differently, and brought too many questions in the beginning, it is likely that I would have been "kicked out" of the opportunity to learn. After studying with my masters in this way for many years, I came to understand that wisdom is born from physical and spiritual experience, and it is possible to find the answers to your own questions through your own practice. I believe my masters trusted that I would continue the legacy of teaching people ways to be self-aware and empowered as they move about the world.

In spiritual cultivation practice, there is a phenomenon called *ZhiShiZhang* 知識障, or "knowledge stagnation." Knowledge stagnation occurs when we over-intellectualize any phenomenon. For instance, we can spend endless hours poring over books and surfing the Internet in order to research Qi 氣. After we have read a certain number of books or studied scores of websites, we may come to think that we have figured it out: "Oh yes, Qi is vital energy. Qi is a concept of ancient Chinese philosophy. Qi is life force. Qi is..." Then, we become Qi-scholars and feel qualified to give lectures on Qi! However, if you focus only on filling your head with other people's ideas of Qi, you hinder your own ability to directly participate in the teachings from Qi itself. Qi is something that can be truly understood only through your own bodily experience. In other words, to learn what Qi is, we must put down our books, turn off our computers, and engage ourselves in Qi-activity. The best way I have found to taste the Qi is to practice NeiGong (traditional Qigong forms) under the guidance of a well-seasoned teacher.

As with my previous book, *Chinese Cosmic Orbit Qigong*, my approach to this book is to follow the wordless tradition. In previous works I have detailed the philosophical roots of Chinese wisdom traditions, so in this book I will focus on sharing the practical perspective of the Fire Dragon Meridian Qigong form from my Mt. Emei 峨嵋 lineage, including relevant bits of background as they relate to the practice itself.

If you are mature NeiGong, Qigong, Taiji, or martial arts practitioners, we believe that practicing this form will help deepen your current understanding of authentic, traditional Chinese internal arts. If you practice the healing arts, we hope that Fire Dragon Meridian Qigong will improve your healing skills and your ability to help others. If you are not yet well acquainted with these traditional Chinese concepts, please do not worry. Whether you are a blossoming Qigong novice or a patient seeking tools for self-healing, you will grow to understand these concepts through your own dedicated practice. For those who are interested in learning more about the philosophical and historical background of traditional Qigong cultivation, you may enjoy reading my book *Vital Breath of The Dao*, or some of my other books published by Singing Dragon.

A Note from Karin

Growing up knowing nature as my temple, I began formalizing my studies of traditional healing arts and eastern philosophies in 1995. I distinctly remember the feeling of palpable relief upon discovering these very ancient and comprehensive methods of understanding that which was already in my soul. It is through my personal cultivation practice that I access my spiraling center— the precious internal compass deep within that allows me to navigate the world with clarity and in service as a naturopathic physician. I bring my dedication as a student of the Dao and my gifts of curiosity, precision, and writing to this work, in hopes that my involvement helps bridge any gaps between the eastern and western mind, so that we all may live with the universal truths of the human heart.

Living with harmonious Qi,

Master Zhongxian Wu
Dr. Karin Taylor Wu

ZheLongKu 蟄龍窟 *(Hibernating Dragon's Den),*
Svarte, Sweden
January 5, 2012

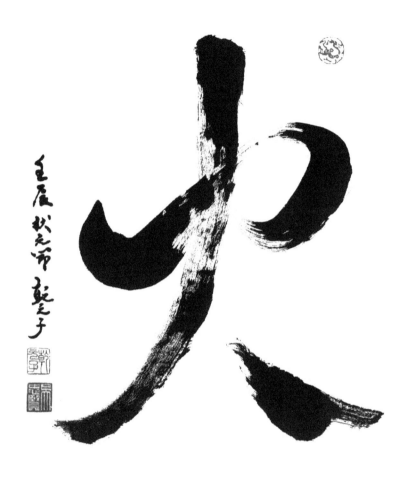

HUO 火—FIRE

1

The Secret of Secrets

ZhiDaGuoZheRuoPengXiaoXian
治大国者若烹小鲜

Ruling a great country is like cooking a small fish

LaoZi, *DaoDeJing*

The Chinese character *Huo* 火 (fire) looks like the dancing flames of a burning fire. It also draws to mind the image of person (*Ren* 人), dripping with sweat. Fire is one of the most important elements, control of which allowed human beings to flourish all over the earth. Fire helps create and sustain new life in the world. According to Chinese Five Phases (aka Five Elements) philosophy, fire was the second element created on earth: After the universe created water, it created fire. The third element created, wood (which represents all new life energy), was generated by the interaction of fire and water. In other words, the earth would be a mass of frozen, lifeless water if not for fire.

In Chinese wisdom traditions, we see the body as a small, microcosmic version of the macrocosmic universe, and the earth herself. As humans, we too will become imbalanced and get sick if we lack fire in our bodies. In fact, we traditionally describe death as the moment fire leaves the body: *HuoJin MingJue* 火盡命絕—when the fire goes out, life ends.

You may be curious about how the fire element is represented inside our bodies. Fire is a symbol for life energy, for our heart-mind, our joy, warmth, and heat. Fire is also the manifestation of our *Shen* 神 or spirit. Through direct observation of nature and a deep awareness of their own bodies, ancient enlightened beings (*Wu* 巫) developed and perfected methods to cultivate their inner fire in order to help them maintain health and achieve enlightenment. Throughout Chinese classical texts and historical documents, these methods are referred to by many different names, such as *DaoYin* 導引 (Guiding Stretch), *TuNa* 吐呐 (Exhale Inhale), *ZuoWang* 坐忘 (Meditate with Emptiness), *NeiDan* 內丹 (Internal Alchemy), *XiuZhen* 修真 (Cultivate Reality), *NeiGong* 內功 (Inner Discipline), *CunSi* 存思 (Visualization), *LianYe* 煉液 (Refine the Fluid), and *NeiGuan* 內觀 (Inner Observation). You may know these methods through their modern and popularized term: Qigong (also spelt Chi-Kung). The term Qigong itself, when referring to a traditional Qigong form, contains the essences captured by its many different names. Throughout this book, we will use the words Qigong and NeiGong interchangeably. Why is this so?

In Chinese, *Nei* means inner, internal, and inside; *Gong* means work, exploit, skill, merit, achievement, and discipline. NeiGong literally means to work internally or to have inner discipline. In other words, by practicing NeiGong we work with our internal subtle energies so that we improve, heighten, and optimize our physical, mental, and spiritual energies. Traditionally, the fundamental practice of NeiGong (Inner Discipline) is that of refining your liquid, *LianYe*. Among all of the historical names of traditional Chinese inner cultivation practices, it is especially important to also understand the meaning of *LianYe*.

Lian 煉 means refine, discipline, practice, exercise, and cultivate. *Ye* 液 means fluid, liquid, water, and *Jing* 精 (essence, in the form of liquid). *Lianye* 煉液 literally translates as "refine your liquid." The first step in refining your liquid is *LianJingHuaQi* 煉精化氣: refining your *Jing* to transform it to Qi. As you may know, *Jing* is the life source and reservoir of your physical body, whereas Qi is the vital energy of your body. The next step in refining your liquid is *LianQiHuaShen* 煉氣化神, or refining your Qi such that it transforms to *Shen* 神, your very spirit. The final step, *LianShenHuanXu* 煉神還虛, is refining your *Shen* to return to *Xu* 虛 (Emptiness). True emptiness is not actually empty but embraces all things—it is the deep spiritual wisdom that informs our daily lives. This process of refining our liquid is akin to the harmonious circulation of water within nature.

With respect to bodily composition of water, the human body mirrors the earth in that it is also made up of about 70 percent water. We look to nature for clues to the behavior and properties of our own internal water cycle. In a frozen environment, there is a paucity of life energy. Solid water (ice) cannot flow and readily nourish vegetation. In warmer, more fiery climates where clean water flows, there is abundance of life. It is in this type of environment that it is easiest to observe the natural cycle of water. Water on the earth (*Jing*, in the form of invisible water vapor from bodies of water, moist ground, and plants) reaches the heavenly sky daily through evaporation. This warm, moisture-laden air (Qi) rises and gathers to form clouds in the heavens (*Shen*). The water droplets present in clouds cool and condense, and rain (our refined *Jing*—our wisdom or "sweet dew") washes down to nourish and replenish the earth (our daily life). As on earth, this cycle of water in our bodies is dependent on the first step—our ability to generate enough inner fire to transform *Jing* to Qi.

Some old Chinese masters like to apply cooking as another analogy to help their students understand this process. In the old days, cooking was not an easy feat. Cooks had no clocks, thermometers, or other modern appliances to control the timing and temperature of their cooking. These primitive conditions were the same as those I grew up with. We needed to perfect our cooking fire by continuously adjusting the wind (a set of bellows) and using our sense and experience in order to make a good meal. Similarly, during a high-level NeiGong or Qigong practice, we refine our *Jing* once we learn how to control our inner fire by utilizing proper breathing techniques.

In our tradition, we liken the body to a nation. You are the emperor or empress of your own great nation. Throughout Chinese history, a great leader was often compared to a great cook—someone who had mastery of fire and the ability to combine the five flavors, yielding a harmonious result to be enjoyed by all. In Chinese cuisine, the five flavors represent all spices. Each spice is classified through the Five Phases/Elements philosophy and can therefore be used specifically to benefit your organ systems. Many Chinese classics use chief, leader, or chef as a metaphor for someone who practices spiritual cultivation. In Chapter 60 of *DaoDeJing,* LaoZi tells us that "ruling a great country is like cooking a small fish." When we cook a delicate fish in the old way, we need to know how to control the cooking fire as well as how to add the right ingredients to make it tasty. Otherwise, we may under- or over-cook the fish, or season it in a way that makes it taste terrible. If the fire gets out of control or if we stop paying attention to it, we run the risk not only of burning the fish, but also of causing a devastating fire disaster. With respect to our spiritual cultivation, conscious beings differentiate themselves by taking great care to safeguard their internal fire. A person or a country's energy resource can be wasted as quickly and easily as carelessly mashing a small fish in the cooking pot if we do not tend it properly.

Chinese culture is a food culture, and learning about food is a way to help us understand Qigong practice and the Dao. In my experience, the traditional way to learn a Qigong form embodies the same methodology we would use to find the prized recipe of a featured dish from a family-owned restaurant.

Although it is not always easy, one can obtain the secret ingredients of a delicious meal from a famous chef. In the old Chinese tradition, different masters held their Qigong and martial arts secrets much like great chefs hold their recipes secret. A master may consent to teach a persevering student some physical movement. The Qigong form itself is the secret ingredient to inner cultivation. However, it is less likely that the master will agree to pass on the knowledge of how to ignite and regulate inner fire. Similarly, if a chef decides to share the secret ingredients of a most famous dish, yet does not disclose the inner secrets of cooking temperature and timing, you could not expect to receive the benefits of the delicious meal. All you would have is a pile of nice ingredients! In Qigong practice, even if you know all the movements, you might never truly savor the richness of the form until the day you are able to master the fire technique. In the higher levels of Qigong practice, the secret of mastering a form is being able to regulate your inner fire—your mental and spiritual focus—by adjusting your wind (the breath). When all of this is done correctly, the perfectly governed body will enjoy a magical, heavenly feast.

I have been teaching Chinese wisdom traditions since 1988, and have had universal feedback of great transformation in health and wellbeing from those who have committed themselves to a daily practice of Fire Dragon Meridian Qigong. Some people have even shared miraculous stories of recovery from advanced cancer after just a few months of dedicated practice. It is the key Qigong form my wife and I offer to people seeking healing from significant, chronic health challenges and traumatic life events. What makes this form so potent? The movements of Fire Dragon Meridian Qigong imitate sparks arising from a bonfire and swirling upward like a spiraling dragon. In addition, the form implements special visualization and breathing techniques that help generate tremendous inner fire. Most of my students, including those in their very first Qigong class or practicing in a freezing cold environment, experience their inner fire during my teaching—often to the point of dripping with sweat. In Fire Dragon Meridian Qigong, we stoke our inner fire and melt away our "ice"—the areas of stagnation, blockage, and disease that reside in our physical, mental, or spiritual bodies. This opens our energetic pathways and allows the smooth flow of Qi in our meridians. Our practice follows the traditional internal alchemy process, where *Jing* (essence) transforms to Qi (vital energy), Qi transforms to *Shen* (spirit), and our *Shen* returns to Emptiness. From Emptiness we access our inner wisdom that reunites our spirit to our physical body.

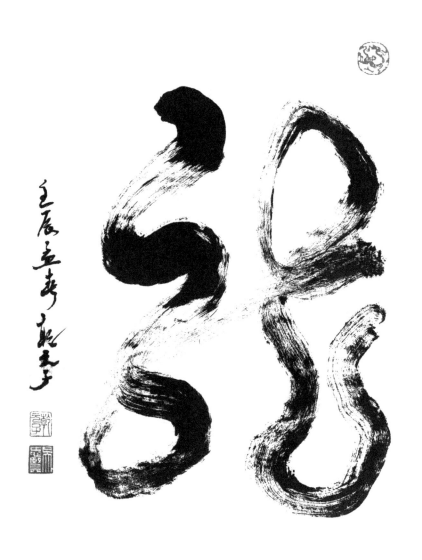

Long 龍—Dragon

2

The Master of Alchemy

YunCongLong
雲從龍

Clouds follow dragon

WEN YAN, *YIJING*

Long 龍, the Chinese dragon, is the legendary and most mystical animal of Chinese culture. In most areas of China, humans themselves are believed to have descended from the dragon. Archeologists have unearthed countless dragon images and icons from ancient China, the oldest one to date from *Liaoning* 遼寧 Province in 1994. There, a great dragon sculpture crafted from seashells has been dated to 6000 BCE. Although prominent in lore since recorded Chinese history, there have been no modern reports of a live dragon sighting as far as we are aware. You may realize that *Long*, the Chinese dragon symbol, holds a different image and spirit than does the western dragon symbol. The body shape of our dragon is long and serpent-like, with four limbs, powerful claws, and no wings. In China, the dragon is not a terrible monster—it is the most auspicious animal. It was the special totem reserved solely for the emperors' use for thousands of years, all the way up until 1911 when the emperor system in

China came to an end. Chinese emperors regarded themselves as True Dragons, the Sons of Heaven.

Dragon represents power, life energy, transformation, communication, connection, freedom, and the universal way. According to Chinese mythology, dragon is the rainmaker, has magic powers that allow it to change natural formations, and can easily fly between heaven and earth. Dragon can penetrate through rock with ease, as dragon makes its home in the rock, just as fish live in water and human beings live in air. If we want to find a dragon, we simply look to the sky. Confucius disclosed the way to seek the dragon in one of his *Ten Wings of Yijing*, *WenYan* 文言: *YunCongLong* 雲從龍, which means that the clouds follow the dragon. The clouds are like the dragons' "groupies," and observing the clouds helps us learn the rich symbolic meaning of dragon on deeper and deeper levels.

In Chinese wisdom traditions, there are many symbolic meanings of dragon. The dragon is the spirit of the East and related to the first life energy, the energy of the Dao itself. It is a symbol for the eastern time of a day (3–9 a.m.) and for the eastern season in the Chinese Lunar–Solar calendar (spring). In China, spring is designated to occur at approximately the same time each year, which according to the Gregorian calendar is the period between February 4 and May 6. In the northern hemisphere, this is the time when nature is in its most magical and transformative season, when new life energy comes forth into the world after a long slumber. Furthermore, dragon represents any time or place when Yang energy (life energy) generates rapid growth and dramatic changes during any new cycle. With respect to the *Yijing*, the tidal hexagram *Guai* 夬 describes the energy of dragon present in our *NeiDan*, or internal alchemy practice.

As discussed in my book *The 12 Chinese Animals*, the Chinese character for *Guai* means decide, dredge, dig, burst, and transform. Hexagram *Guai* is made up of two trigrams. The top trigram is *Dui* 兌 (lake) and the bottom trigram is *Qian* 乾

(heaven). This is an image of a lake over heaven. In *Yijing*, the lake is symbolic of changing old patterns and the transformation from old to new. Heaven exemplifies the continuous orbit of planets as well as the motivation and inner strength it takes to be a great person. Combined, hexagram *Guai* relays an image of great transformation resulting from the unbroken, circulating, and spiraling drive of heaven. *Guai* also bespeaks the transformation that occurs during our internal alchemy practice. When you give witness to the powerful Qi that constantly circulates within your body, you become acutely aware of the great potential for transformation within your body each moment and can feel your mouth fill with aromatic saliva, like a great lake of nectar that nourishes your physical and spiritual bodies.

Dragon is also a symbol for Mother Earth holding her most significant function—to give birth to Ten Thousand Things and to transform them into what they will be. Using our bodies as a microcosmic map of the macrocosmic universe, our belly is our own Mother Earth, and the dragon is hidden within her center, the Lower *DanTian* 丹田. The Lower *DanTian* is located in your lower abdomen and is the center of your life. *DanTian*, which I like to translate as "elixir field," is the place where inner alchemical transformation takes place. In all traditional Chinese internal alchemy cultivation practices, we always emphasize focus on the Lower *DanTian*, especially during our practice. The classics tell us *FengChenZeHua* 逢辰則化—a great transformation is possible only if there is a dragon within.

The Fire Dragon Meridian Qigong form embodies the symbolic power of dragon. Practicing this form is a way to awaken our own hibernating dragons—*ShenQi* 神氣 (spiritual energies); calling upon them helps us transform obstacles in the physical, mental, and spiritual levels. Please join us in cultivating with the master of internal alchemy each day. Together, we will access our own great strength, feel healthier and more vital, gain insight into how to feel our inner peace, and live in harmony with our communities and with Mother Nature.

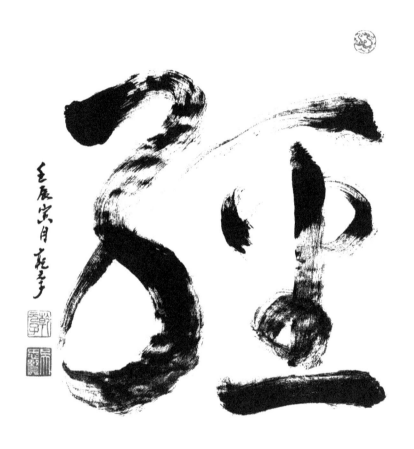

J<small>ING</small> 經—M<small>ERIDIAN</small>

3

The Web of Life

TianWanHuiHui, ShuErBuLo
天网恢恢, 疏而不漏

Heaven's web is vast with a big mesh weave,
yet nothing slips through

LaoZi, *DaoDeJing*

In Chinese, we can use the character *Jing* 經 as a noun, a verb, or an adjective. In general, *Jing* means thread, pass, straight, vertical, longitude, rule, classics, classical, heavenly way, and the meridians of the body. When you spend time learning wisdom traditions from the classical Chinese texts, you may notice that our most important classics are all titled with the same ending character: *Jing*. We see this in the *DaoDeJing* 道德經, *YiJing* 易經, *HuangDi NeiJing* 黃帝內經, *ShiJing* 詩經, etc. We use the same system for identifying those books from foreign languages also written by true enlightened masters. For example, the Bible is called *ShengJing* 聖經, the Torah is known as *TuoLaJing* 妥拉經, our name for the Qur'an is *GuLanJing* 古蘭經, and the Heart and Diamond Sutra are the *XinJing* 心經 and *JinGangJing* 金剛經, respectively. We recognize that truly enlightened masters developed special abilities to cultivate their *Jing* (energy pathways) in order to *Jing* (channel) the secrets of the universe. As such, their teachings and writings themselves are *Jing* (the wisdom from the universe). With respect to our inner cultivation practice, we trust the correct way is to follow those masters' footsteps and work with our *Jing*, the energetic networks within our bodies. In China, we refer to this energy network of our body as the meridian system.

When we dedicate ourselves to practice Qigong daily, we refine our sensitivities so that we are consciously able to experience pathways of flowing Qi in our body. The microcosmic orbit of the body, or the flow of vital energy through our channels and meridians, is responsible for protecting and maintaining the body in a state of health and harmony. If the Qi (vital energy) becomes stagnant or blocked because of an unhealthy lifestyle, destructive attitude, or physical patterns passed to us through our family line, the network as a whole is no longer able to function well. According to Chinese medicine, this kind of stagnation, whether it be found in the physical or mental layers, is the root of all different disease states. In Chapter 10 of *LingShu* 靈樞 (*Spiritual Pivot*), one of the two books of the *HuangDi NeiJing* (*The Yellow Emperor's Classic of Chinese Medicine*), the Yellow Emperor tells us that the meridian system of the body controls a person's life and death, helps heal all kinds of diseases, and can regulate the deficiency and excess of your life energy, allowing Qi to flow freely in your meridian system.

There are many different sizes of meridians in the body. As rivers, streams, and creeks channel the earth's waterways, our meridians weave an invisible energetic web of flowing Qi through our bodies. In addition to the word *Jing* 經, we also use the word *Mai* 脈 when we speak of the meridians. The original meaning of *Mai* refers to the patterns or pulse of flowing water in nature. It is common to use these two characters together, *JingMai* 經 脈, as a compound word for our bodies' meridian systems. In the body, the Twelve Main Meridians and Eight Extraordinary Meridians transport and transform most of the Qi that supports your life and uplifts your spirit. In general, a person will maintain pretty good health throughout their lives if there are no blockages in the Twelve Main Meridians. The Eight Extraordinary Meridians are closed for most adults. If you learn to open these through your inner cultivation practice, you will receive great health and spiritual benefits. In internal alchemy practices, we must learn how to open at least the two most important of the Eight Extraordinary Meridians, the *DuMai* 督脈 and *RenMai* 任脈, in order to achieve the deepest level of Qi and spiritual transformation.

The movements of Fire Dragon Meridian Qigong work with all Twelve Main Meridians and three of the Eight Extraordinary Meridians: the *DuMai*, *RenMai*, and *DaiMai* 帶脈. To help you master the practice, we would like to share a little background knowledge about the meridian system with you:

The Twelve Main Meridians are the pathways of the twelve organ systems and they circulate Qi throughout the whole body. The Qi flow follows certain general patterns within the meridian system:

- *ShouSanYinJing* 手三陰經: The Qi from the three Hand Yin Meridians (Lung, Heart, Pericardium) flows from the chest, runs through the inside of the arms, across the palm, and to the fingertips.

- *ShouSanYangJing* 手三陽經: The Qi from the three Hand Yang Meridians (Large Intestine, Small Intestine, Triple Warmer) flows from the fingertips, up the outside of the arms and across the top of the shoulders to reach the top of the head.

- *ZuSanYinJing* 足三陽經: The Qi from the three Foot Yang Meridians (Bladder, Gallbladder, Stomach) runs from the top of the head, down the back and the back of the legs to the feet.

- *ZuSanYangJing* 足三陰經: The Qi from the three Foot Yin Meridians (Kidney, Liver, Spleen) runs from the feet through inside of your legs and up through the belly to end in the chest.

As you can now imagine, these meridians create a large Qi loop that flows through the whole body. The movements of Fire Dragon Meridian Qigong work with this Qi loop.

In the Eight Extraordinary Meridians, the Chinese character *Mai* is commonly translated as "vessel" in English. For example, *RenMai* is commonly referred to as the "Conception Vessel." Personally, we prefer to use "meridian" consistently when talking about meridians.

DuMai, the Governing Meridian, is located at the center of your back and runs (approximately) along your spine. The Governing Meridian governs all the Yang energy and Yang meridians of your body. If there is no stagnation in your *DuMai* and the Qi can flow freely within it, your Yang energy and inner fire will also flow freely. In this case you will be able to refine and transform the *Jing* to Qi and Qi to *Shen*. Like water transforming from solid to liquid to steam (as we discussed in Chapter 1 of this book), the stagnation that causes disease will melt away into a healthy state of free-flowing Qi.

RenMai, or the Conception Meridian, is located at the center of the trunk of your body and runs (approximately) along your midline. *Ren* 任 means nourish, concept, trust, carry, task, or conception. *RenMai* is the meridian that rules Yin energy and nourishes all Yin meridians of your entire body. Yin energy gives birth to Yang (life) energy, so the *RenMai* also nourishes the Yang energy of your body. Your body will maintain a healthy state and a high level of wellness if your *RenMai* is open, with the Qi flowing smoothly within it.

The *DaiMai* is the Belt Meridian. It is located under the rib cage and, like an invisible belt, it encircles your waist and abdomen. *Dai* 帶 means belt, string, ribbon, bring, carry, hold, or tie. The function of *DaiMai* is to hold all the meridians together in the body, balancing the Qi, blood, and lymph flow between the upper body and lower body. If your belt becomes loose or breaks while you are walking around, you will suddenly find it difficult to move smoothly. Similarly, if your *DaiMai* does not function well, your Qi will not flow well. Some people experience bloating of the belly with a heavy feeling in the waist and legs when this happens. For women, *DaiMai* problems often manifest as an unhealthy vaginal discharge.

In Fire Dragon Meridian Qigong, we consider these fifteen meridians as the key links that connect everything in our body to our *DanTian* (elixir field), weaving together a strong web of health, happiness, and harmony throughout our lives.

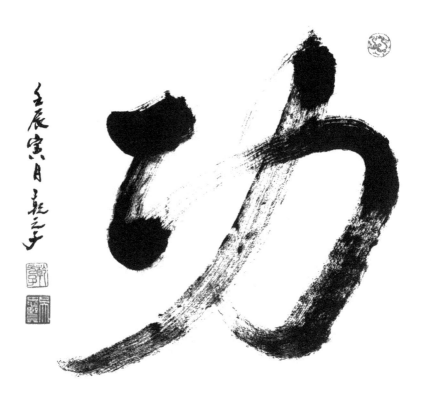

GONG 功—QIGONG

4

The Journey to All Wonders

XuanZhiYouXuan, ZhongMiaoZhiMen
玄之又玄, 眾妙之門

Mystery of mysteries, the doorway of all wonders

Laozi, *DaoDeJing*

Gong is the abbreviated name for *NeiGong*, which was later replaced by the term *Qi*Gong. The modern, popularized term Qigong refers to a traditional Chinese way of life—living in health and harmony with community and nature through physical, mental, and *Shen* (spiritual) cultivation. At its essence, Qigong is a method of Qi cultivation that has been used for thousands of years. Qi cultivation brings about a deep inner awareness and creates the foundation for health and a state of conscious being that allows you to experience inner peace in your life, shifting and transforming turbulent emotional states with ease.

As discussed in my book *The Vital Breath of the Dao*, the Chinese character *Gong* 功 contains the radical *Gong* 工 and the radical *Li* 力. *Gong* 工 means labor, project, skill, delicate, result, work, and worker. The original meaning of *Gong* 工 was a carpenter's square, the tool of a highly skilled artisan who could understand and utilize precision to create a work of beauty and perfection. As such, it symbolizes the laws of the universe. The original meaning of the *Li* 力 radical is a tendon in the body, and it implies using all one's best, whether that be force, power, effort, or strength. Therefore, *Gong* 功 creates an image of a person following a precise path, putting forth his (or her) best effort to improve his Qigong skill. To make sure we are following the way properly, we set out to find an illuminated teacher and follow her (or his) instruction precisely in order to receive the full benefits of our Qigong practice.

Reflecting the three layers that construct the universe—*Tian* 天 (heaven), *Di* 地 (earth), and *Ren* 人 (human being)—traditional training in Qigong also emphasizes three layers: the physical body, the Qi or energy body, and the spiritual body. Your whole body has these three layers, as does each part of your body. For example, your finger is not just a simple finger, but has three parts—the physical component, the energetic component, and the spiritual component. This is the same for each part of your body—your hair, your eye, your knee, your heart, etc. The body is a microcosm of the macrocosmic universe, and the three layers of the body (as a whole and all of its parts) are the same as the three layers of the universe—*Jing*, Qi, and *Shen*, which we have translated for you previously as Essence, Vital Energy, and Spirit.

We always work with *Jing*, Qi, and *Shen* during our personal cultivation practice and during our healing work. We regard them as our Three Treasures—they are highest form of medicine for all human beings. Next, we will provide a little more detail about the three layers of our body.

The *Jing* Layer: Healing

Jing (essence) represents the physical body in Chinese wisdom traditions. The physical body contains our essential life energy. From the *Jing* perspective, you will notice your physical body start to change and grow stronger with your Qigong practice. Some patients recover from disease just by going through training of the body alone.

No matter what, it is a good idea to strengthen our physical bodies—our physical body holds our Qi body and our spiritual body. If we are sick or otherwise debilitated, it can be more challenging to sit or stand for long periods of time during our spiritual cultivation practice. Thus, the foundation of Qigong practice involves healing the physical body and building up our health and stamina so that we can withstand the rigors of deeper levels of cultivation.

The keystone of working with *Jing* is correct posture. In traditional Chinese spiritual cultivation or martial arts training, we always emphasize practicing with the correct physical posture. The correct posture is a model of life. With the right bearing, we can easily overcome obstacles and resist chronic illness. With correct posture, our Qi is able to circulate and flow naturally, without stagnation. Healing is a direct result of this free-flowing circulation. Also, when your energy is strong and free-flowing, you can use your Qigong skills to transmit your energy to help others.

The Qi Layer: Transforming

In Chinese, Qi has many meanings. In inner cultivation, Qi means life energy and is the vital energy of the body. Qi can also be translated as "vital breath." At the Qi layer of Qigong training, we focus how to strengthen *Jing* and transform it to Qi, and then how to refine Qi and transform it to *Shen*. The heart of this practice is the breath.

Life is within the breath. We utilize special breathing techniques, like breathing with our skin, as ways to control our inner fire. By controlling our inner fire we are able to make great transformation in our bodies and in our lives. Traditional Qigong forms draw upon many different breathing methods to help shift various blockages in the physical, mental, and spiritual levels.

Through the breath, the Qigong practitioner learns to work with and release disease by using the Qi itself to work out areas of stagnation and to transform pathogenic (disease-causing) factors. This principle is similar to the one we use when facing a martial arts opponent. When we allow ourselves to enter into a Qi state and understand the flow of Qi, we can quickly and effortlessly shift our energy so that we master our opponent without fighting or struggle.

If you can pay close attention to your breath, deepening and slowing down your breathing throughout your daily life, you will be more in touch with this Qi state. By maintaining awareness of your breath you will discover a powerful way to increase your vital energy and life force. A cultivated Qi body will always help you find ways to navigate around all obstacles with minimal effort.

The *Shen* Layer: Flowing

Shen (spirit) is a term used to describe the spiritual body. In general, our mind is related to our *Shen*. Once we pay too much attention to the external world, or worry too much about what's going on in our lives, we run the risk of disturbing our spiritual body. If we always look outside ourselves, we will leak our *ShenQi* 神氣 (spiritual energy). To prevent this leakage, we must be sure to bring our eyesight back to our body and look within during our cultivation practice. In Qigong terminology, this practice is called *ShenGuang HuiShou* 神光回收. *ShenGuang* means spiritual light and eyesight while *HuiShou* means return back or pull back. By closing our eyes and bringing our awareness within, we bring our spiritual light back to our body.

Our mind, thoughts, and attitudes are all related to our spiritual body. When we cultivate at this level of practice, we access the sage that resides in our heart-minds by looking within and regulating our spiritual light. In traditional Qigong forms, we look within and use different visualization techniques to regulate our heart-mind and awaken our spirit and inner wisdom. True enlightenment stems from living our heart's truth. When we practice at the *Shen* level, we cultivate deep compassion for ourselves, allowing that compassion to spill over to others, and we focus on *TianRenHeYi* 天人合一, or living with the flow of nature or Dao.

Fire Dragon Meridian Qigong form is an ancient method of transforming areas of stagnation in all layers of our bodies. Practicing every day will strengthen and balance your body, mind, and spirit. Through the practice, you will be able to bring your three best medicines—*Jing*, Qi, and *Shen*—together to exist in harmony. In doing so, we strengthen our life energy, release stagnation, transform disease, and move closer to the Dao and immortality.

From the viewpoint of Daoist practitioners, Daoism is the tradition of immortality, meaning that the journey of Daoist cultivation practices is one towards immortality. This often begs the question of what exactly is meant by immortality. The idea of immortality or everlasting life has nothing to do with yearning to live forever. The ancient Daoist master ZhuangZi 莊子 (also translated as Chuang Tzu) stated in *QiWuLun* 齊物論:

> *MoShouYuShangZi, ErPengZuWeiYao.*
> 莫寿于殇子，而彭祖为夭

> There is no life longer than that of a child who has died in infancy, while the 800-year-old sage, PengZu 彭祖 died young.

On a superficial level, of course no living being can escape death. Death is simply a part of the Five Elements' cycle of the universe. At the same time, a process of rebirth always follows death, and thus, there is no such thing as absolute, isolated death.

In the Immortal's tradition, we have an expression, *XinSi ShenHuo* 心死神活, which translates as "allow your heart to die so that your spirit will live." We have interpreted this to mean that by embracing death and bringing it gracefully into our hearts, we will truly understand the knowledge of immortality. In Chinese, the word for immortal is *Xian* 仙, which is a pictograph of a person who lives on a mountain. Throughout history, many Daoist masters have referred to themselves as *ShanRen* 山人— Mountain People—because they spend long periods living as hermits in the mountains, cultivating their heart-mind. Another word for immortal is *ZhenRen* 真人—real or true human being. From the Chinese ideogram, we see that the concept of an immortal is of one who has cultivated good health, happiness, and humanity and embodies these qualities in everyday life. We hope the Fire Dragon will help you live with the wisdom and grace of your own immortality.

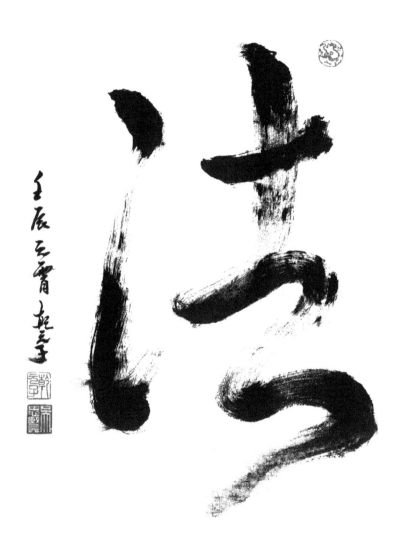

_Fa_ 法—THE PRACTICE

Fire Dragon Meridian Qigong

The general image of this form, as depicted by the names of each movement, is that of pure potential hidden deep within, rising from the depths of winter slumber and bursting forth with new life energy. Although there is rich *Yijing* symbolism behind the names of each movement of the Fire Dragon Meridian Qigong form, we will not address them in this book. With respect to ancient Chinese wisdom traditions, we firmly believe that some subtle teachings are properly transmitted in person.

5.1

QianLongYinZhen
乾龍隱真

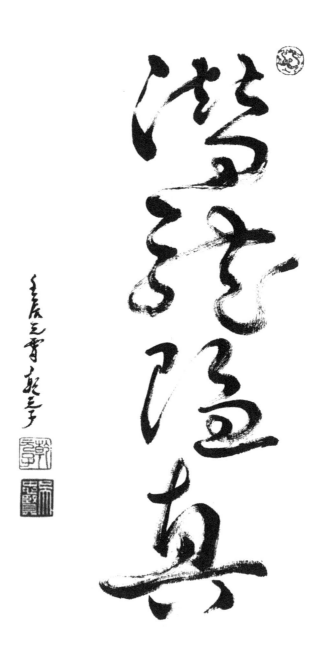

Dragon Hides the Treasure

Movement

Stand with your feet together with your toes grabbing the earth. Straighten your neck and keep your head upright. Relax your body, from the top of your head to the bottom of your feet. Imagine the top of your head touches heaven, and that the *Tianmen* 天門 (or "Heavenly Gate/GV20"—an acupuncture point on the top of your head) is open. Straighten your back so that it feels as solid as a mountain. Make sure to relax and drop your shoulders in order to open your chest. In Chinese wisdom traditions, your chest is related to your heart. Open your heart. Keep your arms hanging naturally by your sides, with your fingers straight yet relaxed. Lift your perineum to seal *Dihu* 地戶 (or "Earthly Door/CV1"—an acupuncture point located in the tissue between your anus and your sexual organs). Tuck in your lower abdomen. Place the tip of your tongue on the roof of your mouth, specifically on the tooth ridge behind your upper teeth, and make the "Magpie Bridge" (*QueQiao* 鵲橋). Please remember your *DuMai* and *RenMai*, the two important acupuncture meridians that run along your midline in the front and back of your body. These meridians disconnect at the roof of your mouth. When we make the Magpie Bridge, we connect these two meridians, helping the Qi to flow smoothly in our bodies.

Keep your teeth closed and your mouth closed. Relax your eyelids (*ShenGuangHuiShou* 神光回收) and bring your eyesight and spiritual light back to your body. Look within. Listen within. Breathe with your nose, with your lungs, and with all the pores of your skin. Open all the pores of your body and allow the Qi, like sunlight, to pour into your body through your skin. Imagine the Qi condensing into your *DanTian* 丹田, the "elixir field" in your lower belly.

Feel your body merging with the Qi through each breath. Adjust your breathing to be slow, smooth, deep, and even. Your breath should be soundless. In Chinese, this breathing technique is called *MiMi MianMian* 密密綿綿, meaning breath that is soft and unbroken like cotton and silk. (Figure 1)

Function

At first glance, this movement seems easy to follow. From an external point of view, it almost appears as though you are doing nothing. In fact, this movement embodies the fundamental elements of every traditional Chinese cultivation practice. Each element of this posture is designed to preserve your Qi and recharge your life energy.

Daily practice of this movement will help you recover from a state of weakness, strengthening your vitality by building up your internal Qi, and bring balance and clarity to your heart-mind. It is a way to help you directly experience your Three Treasures (the healing powers hidden deep within your body), awaken your consciousness, and replenish your *Yuan Qi* 元氣, the source of your life energy. This movement opens your body, enables you to connect with the universal Qi, and evokes your spirit. Regular practice of this standing form is the cornerstone of healing, harmony, and spiritual cultivation.

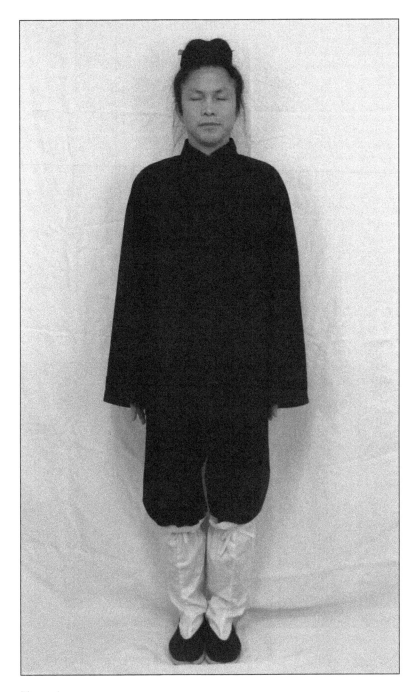

Figure 1

5.2

LongXianYuTian

龍見於田

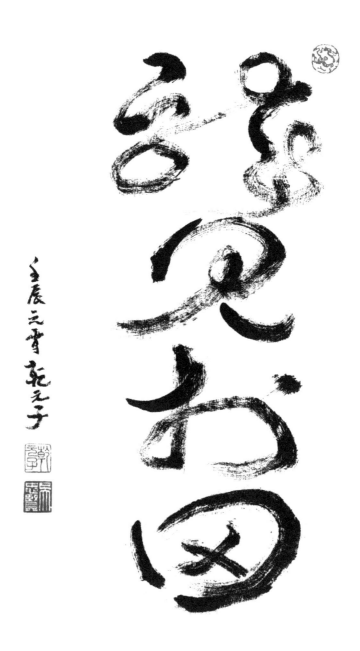

Dragon Appears on the Field

Movement

With your arms still hanging in a relaxed way by your sides, make sure your fingers are straight. Extend your fingers far away. Imagine that your fingers are penetrating deep into the earth. Merge your Qi with the earthly Qi. With your inhale, slowly bring your hands up along the sides of your body. With your fingers, draw the earthly Qi up from the center of the earth. (Figure 2)

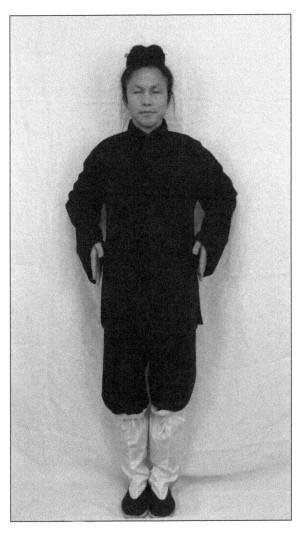

Figure 2

Once you reach the level of your waist, exhale and slowly bend your wrists so that your palms face heaven and your fingers point towards your Belt Meridian. Allow the earthly Qi to flow from your fingertips into your *DanTian* through your Belt Meridian. Feel the Qi connecting through your body between your fingertips. (Figure 3)

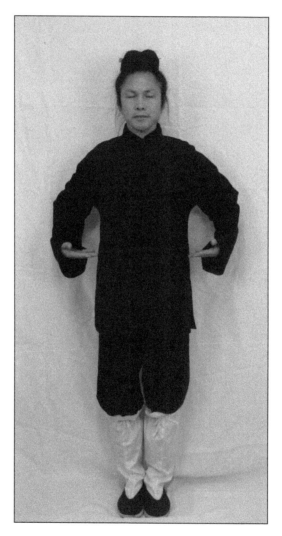

Figure 3

Next, take a deep breath. With your next exhalation, rotate your hands forward, one finger at a time, as you extend your forearms in front of you. With your palms facing heaven and your elbows bent and close to your waist, your forearms are now parallel with the earth. Extend your fingers far away and feel them touching the end of the universe. Merge your Qi with the universal Qi. (Figures 4, 4a)

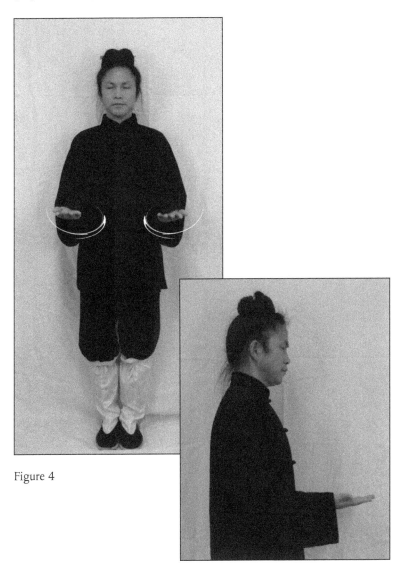

Figure 4

Figure 4a

Inhale and turn your fingers inward, one by one, so that they point towards your navel. Visualize sending universal Qi into your *DanTian* through your fingertips. (Figure 5)

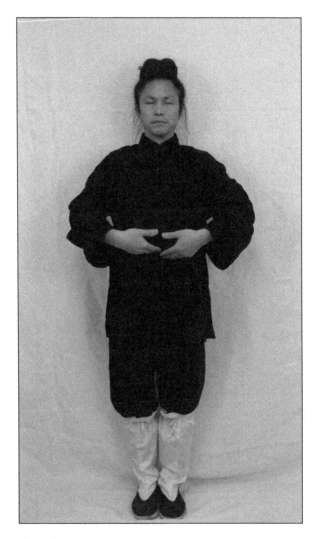

Figure 5

Exhale as you continue turning your hands so that your palms now face your lower belly and make a triangle with your thumbs and index fingers. Pour the Qi into your *DanTian*. (Figure 6)

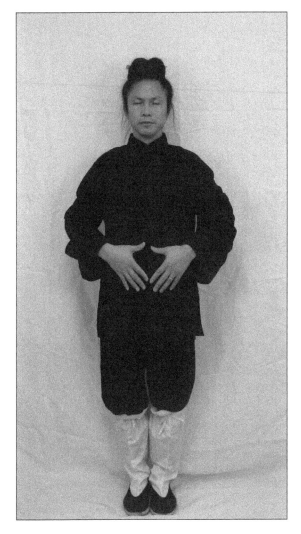

Figure 6

Circle your hands over your *DanTian*. Inhale as you complete one half circle and exhale as you complete the other half of the circle. Circle your *DanTian* counterclockwise three times and then clockwise three times. (Figures 6a, 6b, 6c)

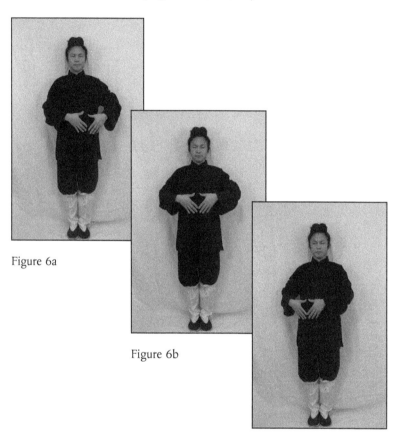

Figure 6a

Figure 6b

Figure 6c

Function

Regular practice of *LongXianYuTian* will help build up your earthly Qi and optimize your digestive function. It is also a good technique for those of you who are seeking methods to strengthen weakened muscles, tendons, or ligaments. People who do healing work will notice that their ability to help others will be significantly increased after just a few months of daily practice.

5.3

LongYueZaiYuan
龍躍在淵

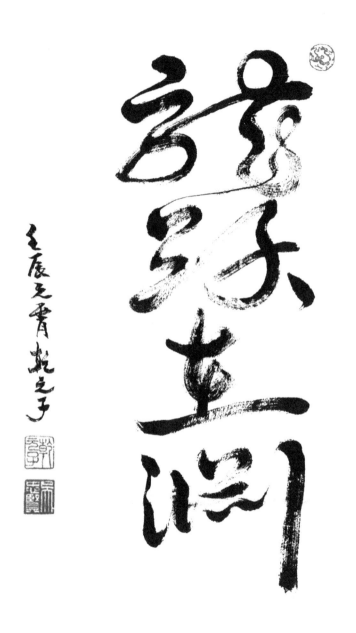

Dragon Leaps out of the Abyss

Movement

Turn your palms up, with your fingertips pointing towards each other. (Figure 7) Take a deep breath, imagine opening all the pores of your skin to allow the universal Qi to enter into your *DanTian*, and raise your hands to the level of your middle *DanTian* (located near the center of your chest) as you lift your heels. (Figures 7a, 7b)

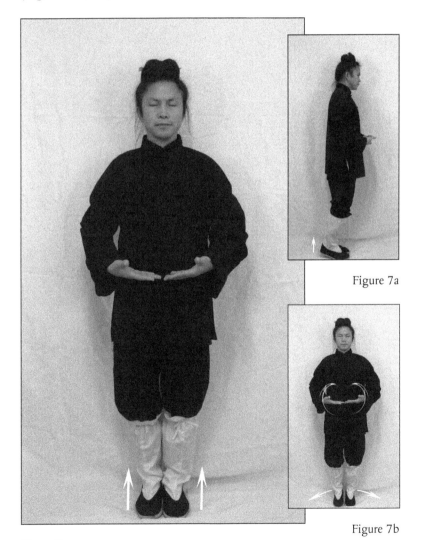

Figure 7a

Figure 7b

Figure 7

Holding your breath, flip your palms down to face earth and turn the heels of your feet out so that your knees point toward each other. (Figure 8) Gently place your heels back down on the earth as you bring your hands back down to your *DanTian*. (Figure 8a)

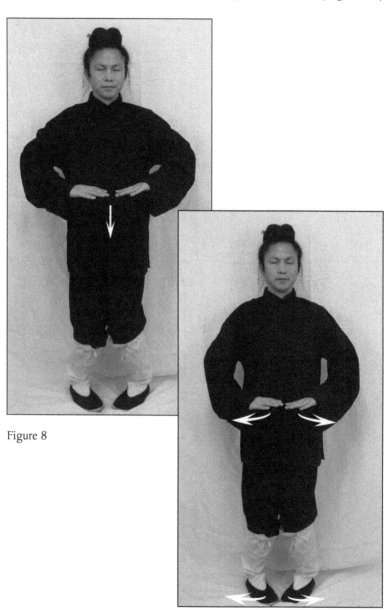

Figure 8

Figure 8a

As you exhale, turn your fingers outwards, one by one, and move your arms in a slight arc to rest in front of your body. Your forearms are parallel to the earth, with palms facing down, and your elbows are bent and close to your waist. Stop when your arms reach about a 45-degree angle from your center and extend your fingers far away to gather the universal Qi. While you are opening your arms, also turn your toes out, pointing your knees away from each other. (Figure 9)

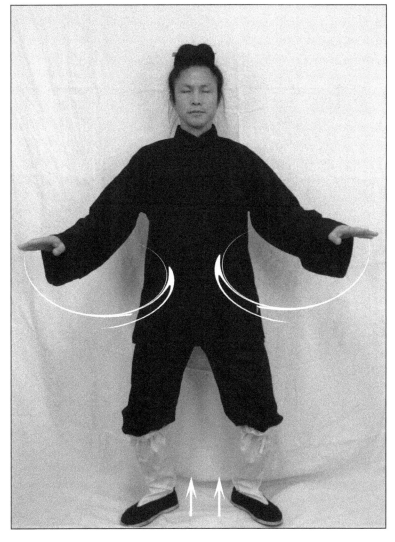

Figure 9

Repeat the above movement twice more, so that you come to rest standing in a wide horse stance. (Figures 10, 10a, 10b, 10c) At the end of the third sequence, make sure your feet are parallel to each other, with toes pointing forward and grabbing the earth. Your knees will be slightly bent, with your lower legs stable and upright like the sturdy trunk of a tree. Please note that it is very important to make sure that your knees never extend beyond your toes.

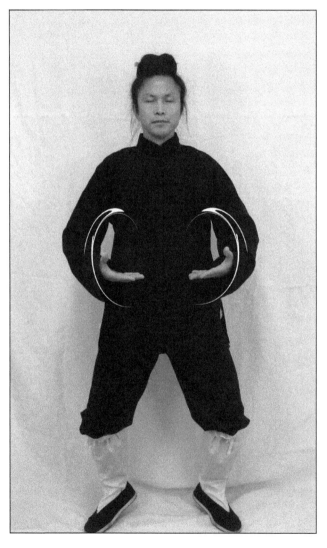

Figure 10

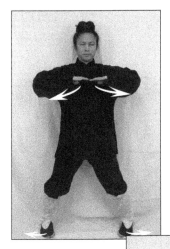

Figure 10a

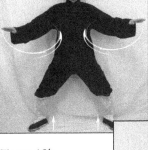

Figure 10b

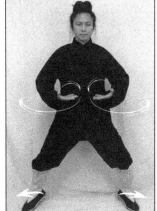

Figure 10c

On your inhale, move your hands toward your *DanTian* and imagine scooping the universal Qi back to your body. (Figure 11)

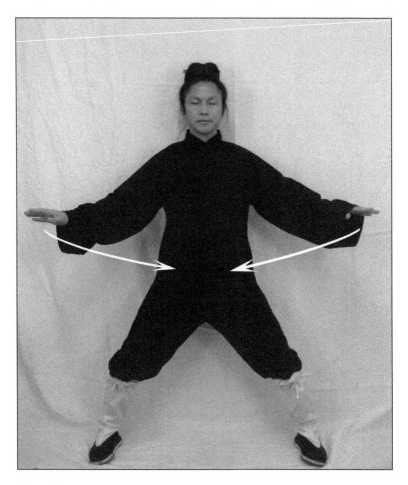

Figure 11

Exhale and bring your hands in to rest over your *Dan Tian*.
Visualize pouring the universal Qi into your *Dan Tian*. With your
palms facing your *Dan Tian*, focus on your *Dan Tian*. (Figure 12)

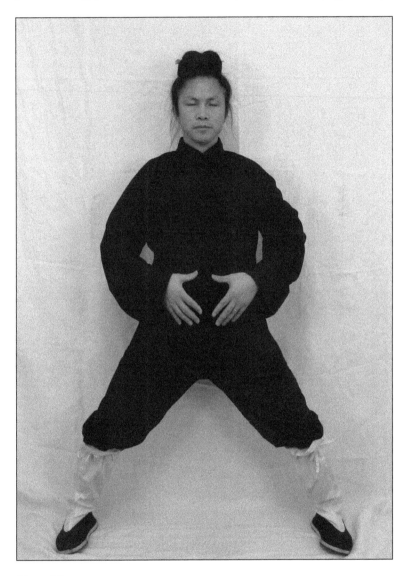

Figure 12

Function

The hands and feet are the most distal parts of your body, being the furthest away from the organs in your center. It requires effort for your organs to transport their Qi through the Twelve Main Meridians to reach your hands and feet. Your hands and feet also act as "U-turn" points where the meridians of your Yin and Yang organs meet and switch over towards each other. *LongYueZaiYuan* focuses on working with these pivotal areas to ensure proper Qi circulation through your Twelve Main Meridians, thus helping energy flow freely throughout your whole body.

5.4

LongZhanYuYe
龍戰於野

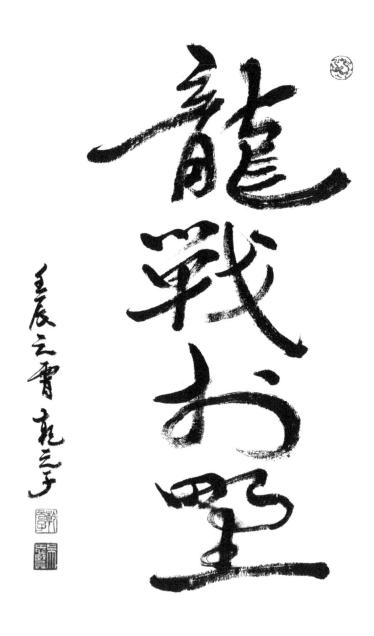

Dragon Battles on the Field

Movement

The Rising Dragon: Slowly raise your arms up your midline. Move your left arm slightly outward so that it is rounded in a full arc in front (slightly off center) of your body at shoulder height and the right arm is rounded closer in towards your body at the level of the center of your chest. Both palms should be facing your body. Next, spiral your hands, wrists, and arms with a spiraling motion that originates from your *DanTian*. Feel your entire body whorl like a rising dragon. (Figures 13, 13a)

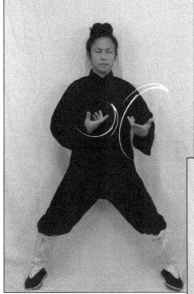

Figure 13

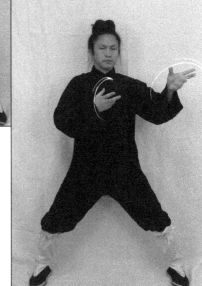

Figure 13a

Tapping Left Hand Yin Meridians: With strong fingers and a loose wrist, tap the left-sided three Hand Yin Meridians with your right hand. Starting from the center of your chest, tap through the inside of your left arm all the way to your palm and left fingertips. Imagine that you are penetrating universal Qi from your right fingers into the meridians as you tap. When you finish, the left palm will be facing you and the right palm will face away from your body. (Figures 14, 14a, 14b, 14c)

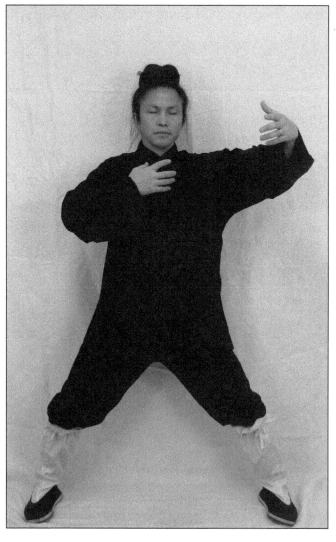

Figure 14

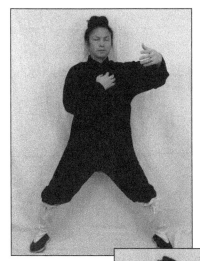

Figure 14a

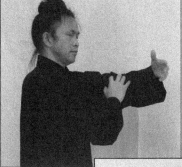

Figure 14b

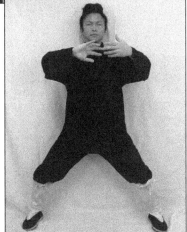

Figure 14c

Embracing the Pearl: Slowly turn over your left hand so that both palms face away from your body. With your fingers pointing towards each other, stretch your hands. Reach your pinky fingers towards heaven and extend your thumbs into the earth. (Figure 15)

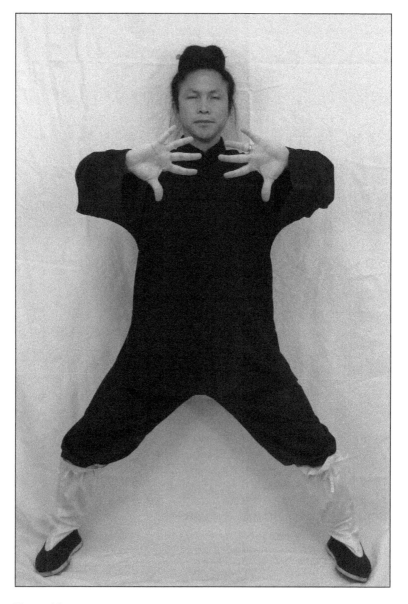

Figure 15

Feel the Qi connection between your hands. Continue to feel this connection as you pull your arms open to your side. With your palms facing away from you, open your chest. (Figure 16)

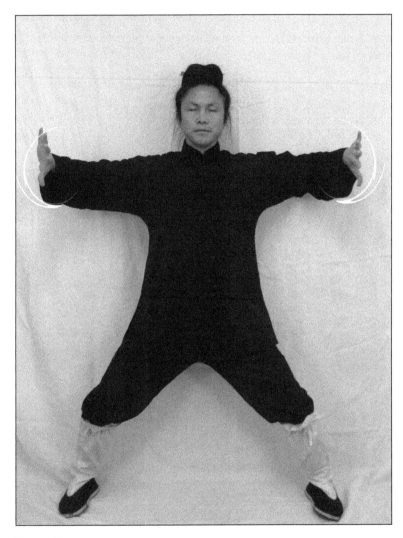

Figure 16

Next, rotating from your shoulders, turn your palms to face your body and embrace the Qi. Inhale and imagine you are holding a big ball of Qi. (Figure 17)

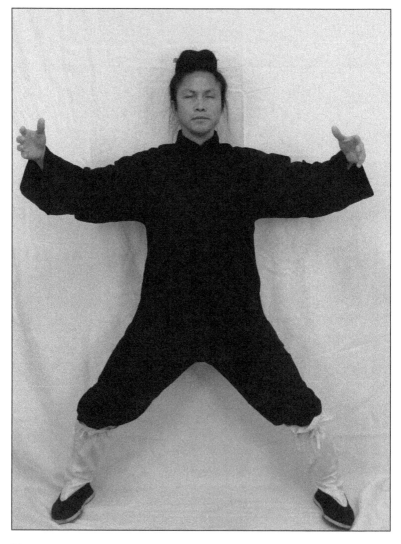

Figure 17

Exhale and bring your hands together with a forceful clap. (Figure 18)

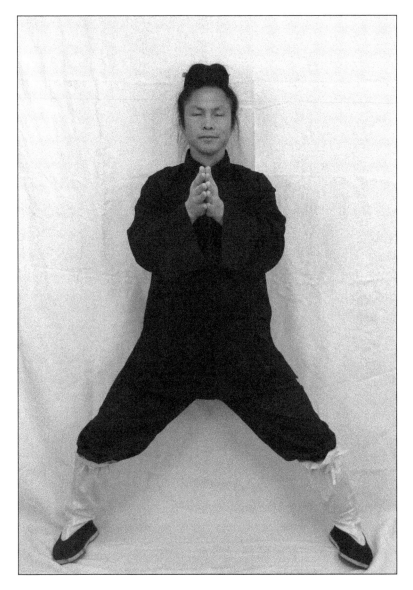

Figure 18

Inhale and gracefully open your arms again to embrace the Qi. (Figure 19)

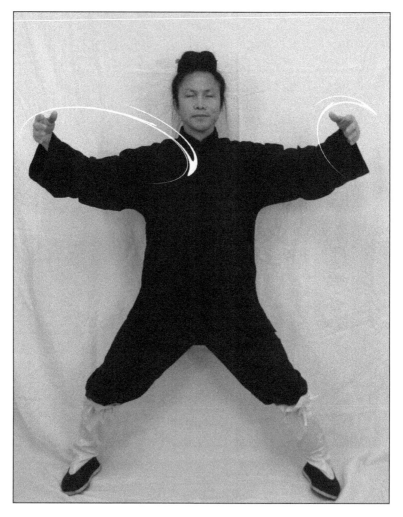

Figure 19

Turning Heaven and Earth: Open your left arm about 45 degrees from your body with your left palm facing heaven. Feel your left hand connecting with heaven. At the same time, bend your right elbow and bring your right palm, facing earth, closer to your body at the level of your chest. Feel your right hand connecting with the earth. (Figure 20)

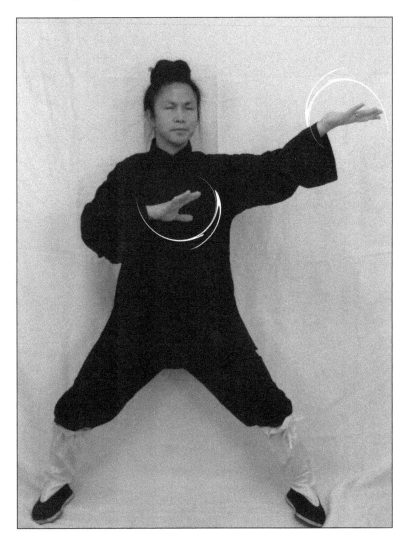

Figure 20

Spiral your hands one finger at a time so that your left palm now faces earth and your right palm faces heaven. (Figure 21)

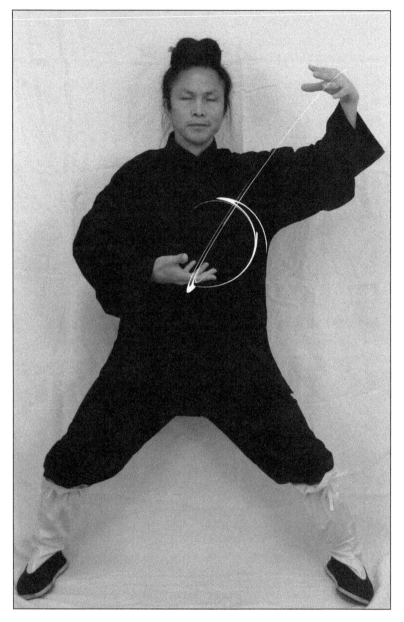

Figure 21

Bend your left arm, bringing your left hand to your chest, palm still facing earth. At the same time, rotate your right hand so that it now hovers, palm facing earth, directly over top of the left hand. (Figure 22)

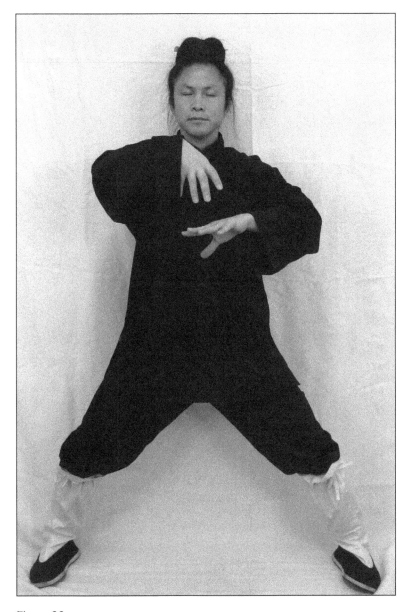

Figure 22

Tapping Left Hand Yang Meridians: With your right hand, tap your Left Hand Yang Meridians. With strong fingers and a loose wrist, tap from your left fingers up along the outside of the left arm (Figure 23), across the top of the left shoulder, up the side of your neck and to the top of your head. Imagine that you are penetrating universal Qi from your right fingers into the meridians as you tap. At the same time, the left hand gradually moves downward until it reaches the level of your *DanTian*, with left palm facing earth. Imagine pouring heavenly Qi into your Heavenly Gate on top of your head through your right hand. (Figure 23a)

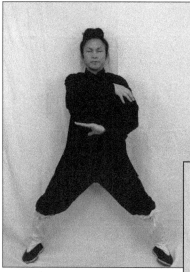

Figure 23

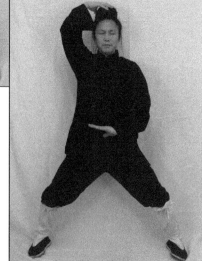

Figure 23a

The Rising Dragon: Rotate your right wrist, with the pinky finger moving around your ear and over the top to your shoulder to face forward, ending with the thumb by your ear. (Figures 24) Continue to move your right fingers away from you while extending your right arm. (Figure 24a)

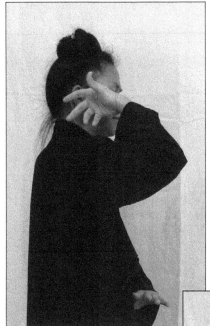

Figure 24

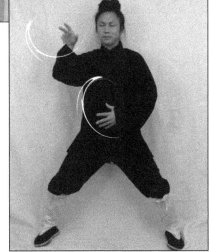

Figure 24a

As your right arm is extending away from you at shoulder height, spiral your left hand upwards from your *DanTian* to the level of your chest. Rotate your hands, wrists, and arms with a spiraling motion that originates from your *DanTian*. Feel your entire body whorl like a rising dragon. (Figure 25)

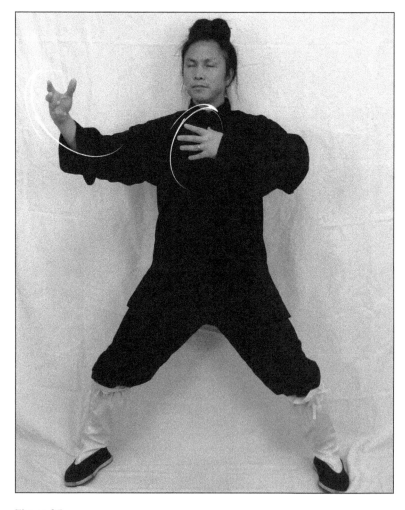

Figure 25

Tapping Right Hand Yin Meridians: With strong fingers and a loose wrist, tap the right-sided three Hand Yin Meridians with your left hand. Starting from the center of your chest, tap through the inside of your right arm all the way to your palm and right fingertips. (Figure 26) Imagine that you are penetrating universal Qi from your left fingers into the meridians as you tap. When you finish, the right palm will be facing you and the left palm will face away from your body. (Figure 26a)

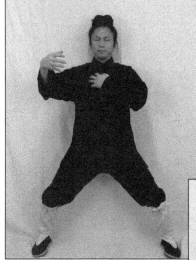

Figure 26

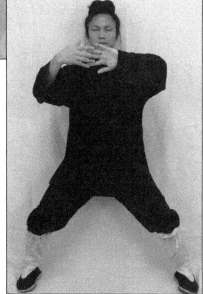

Figure 26a

Embracing the Pearl: Slowly turn over your right hand so that both palms face away from your body. With your fingers pointing towards each other, stretch your hands. Reach your pinky fingers towards heaven and extend your thumbs into the earth. (Figure 27)

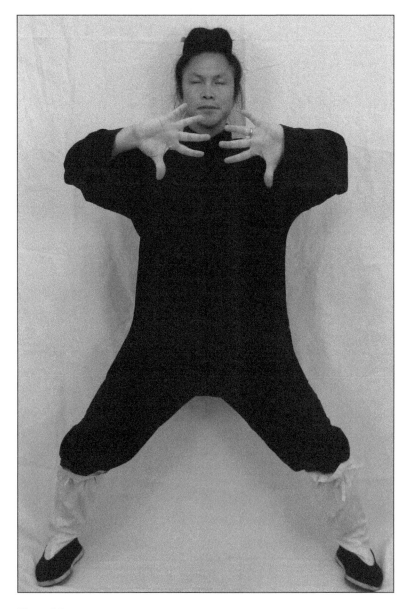

Figure 27

Feel the Qi connection between your hands. Continue to feel this connection as you pull your arms open to your side. With your palms facing away from you, open your chest. (Figure 28)

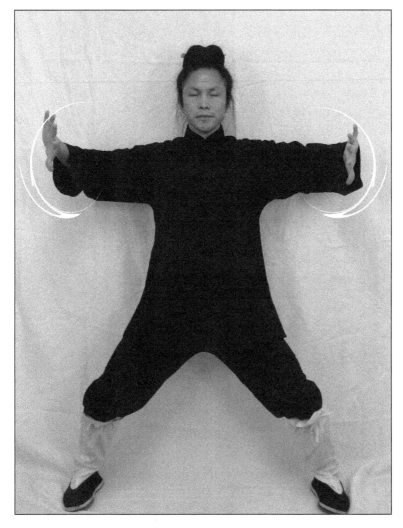

Figure 28

Next, rotating from your shoulders, turn your palms to face your body and embrace the Qi. Inhale and imagine you are holding a big ball of Qi. (Figure 29)

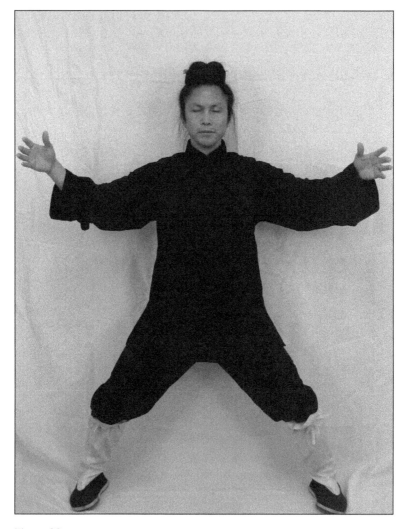

Figure 29

Exhale and bring your hands together with a forceful clap. (Figure 30)

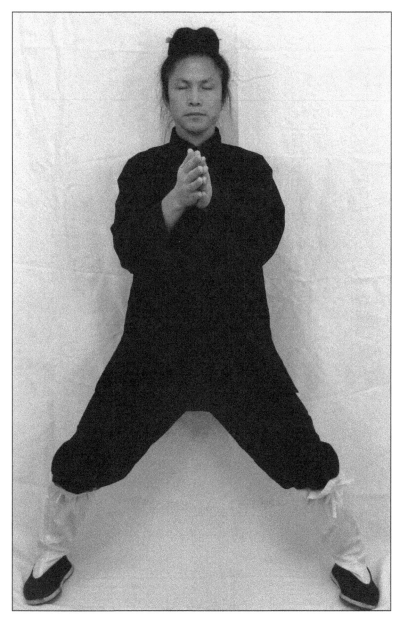

Figure 30

Inhale and gracefully open your arms to embrace the Qi again. (Figure 31)

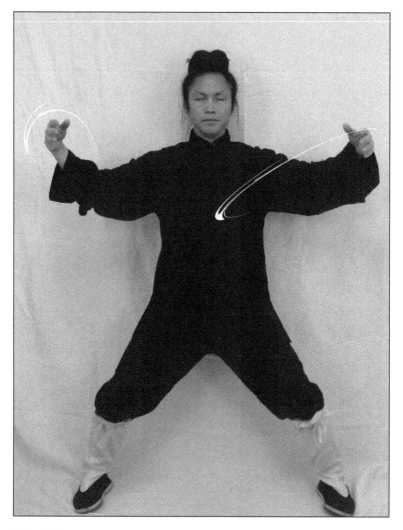

Figure 31

Turning Heaven and Earth: Open your right arm about 45 degrees from your body, with your right palm facing heaven. Feel your right hand connecting with heaven. At the same time, bend your left elbow and bring your left palm, facing earth, closer to your body at the level of your chest. Feel your left hand connecting with the earth. (Figure 32)

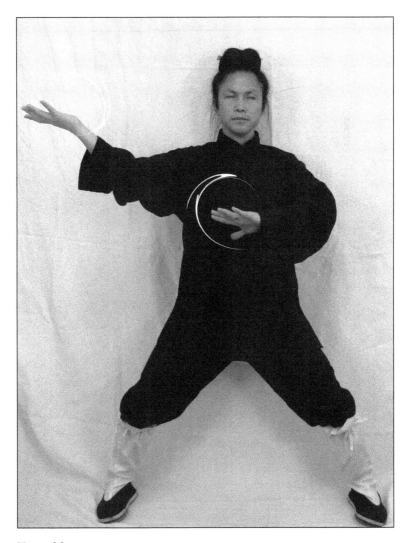

Figure 32

Spiral your hands one finger at a time so that your right palm now faces earth and your left palm faces heaven. (Figure 33)

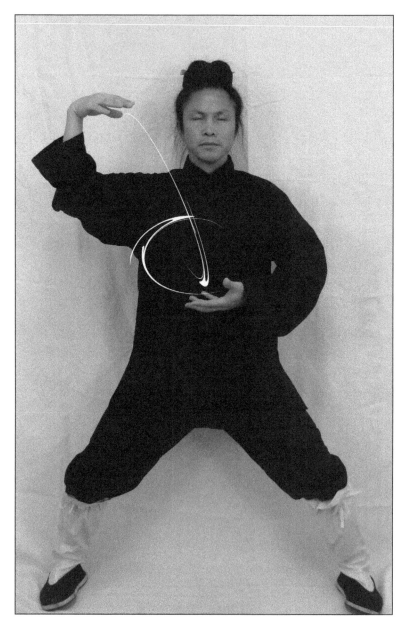

Figure 33

Bend your right arm, bringing your right hand to your chest, palm still facing earth. At the same time, rotate your left hand so that it now hovers, palm facing earth, directly over top of the right hand. (Figure 34)

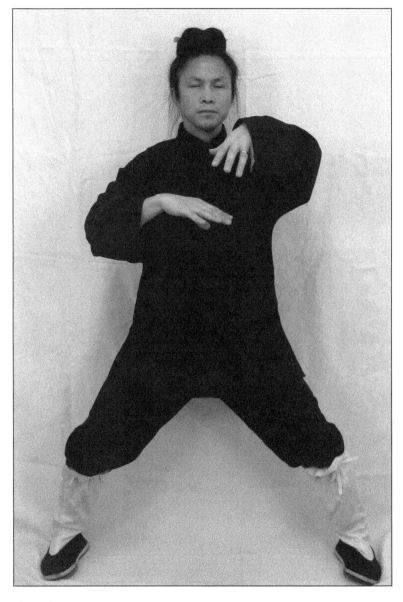

Figure 34

Tapping Right Hand Yang Meridians: With your left hand, tap your Right Hand Yang Meridians. With strong fingers and a loose wrist, tap from your right fingers up along the outside of the right arm (Figure 35), across the top of the right shoulder, up the side of your neck and to the top of your head. Imagine that you are penetrating universal Qi from your left fingers into the meridians as you tap. At the same time, the right hand gradually moves downward until it reaches the level of your Lower *DanTian*, with right palm facing earth. Imagine pouring heavenly Qi into your Heavenly Gate on top of your head through your left hand. (Figure 35a)

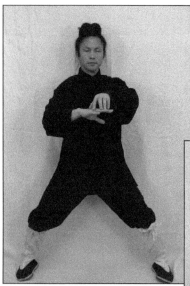

Figure 35

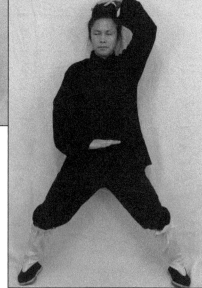

Figure 35a

Taking a Qi Shower: Rotate your left hand down, with your pinky side moving along your left ear toward your left shoulder so that your left palm is cupped over your shoulder, close to your ear. (Figure 36) Swing your right arm up to reach the sky. (Figure 36a)

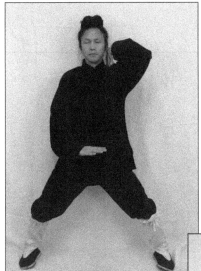

Figure 36

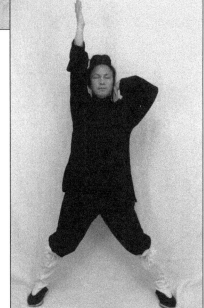

Figure 36a

Rotate your right fingers to grasp the heavenly Qi and bring your right hand, cupped, down to your right shoulder, close to your ear. Pour the Qi into your body through the top of your shoulders. Feel as though you are taking a Qi shower. (Figure 37)

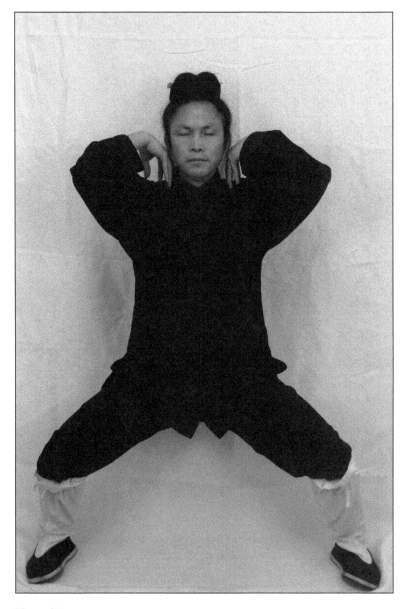

Figure 37

Next, squat down, as low as you can, while keeping your back straight. (Figure 38) In a squatting position, rotate your palms so that they face outward. Your hands are close to your ears and your fingers are pointing towards heaven. (Figure 38a)

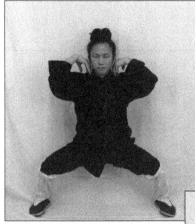

Figure 38

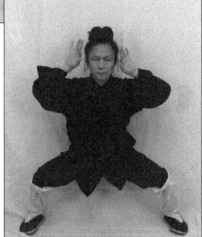

Figure 38a

Straighten your legs and arms. Reach up with your fingertips and touch the heavens. Stretch and open one side of your body, then the other, alternating left and right. Imagine you are a dragon flying the sky. (Figure 39)

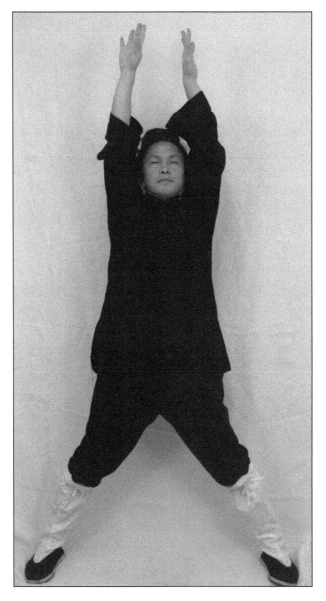

Figure 39

Rotate your hands to gather the heavenly Qi. (Figure 40) Lower your Qi-filled hands so they rest above the top of your head. Pour the Qi into your body through your Heavenly Gate. Feel as though you are taking a Qi shower. (Figure 40a)

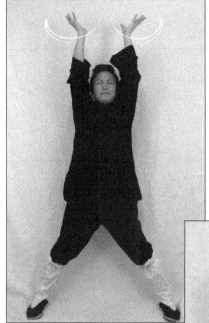

Figure 40

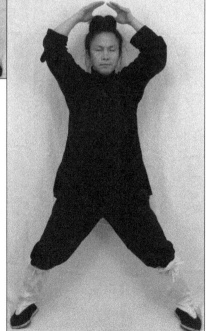

Figure 40a

Tapping the Foot Yang Meridians: Next, bring your hands to the top of your head and begin tapping your three Foot Yang Meridians. With strong fingertips and a loose wrist, tap the top of your head, the back of your head, your neck, and your upper back. (Figures 41, 41a)

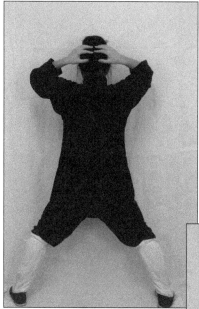

Figure 41

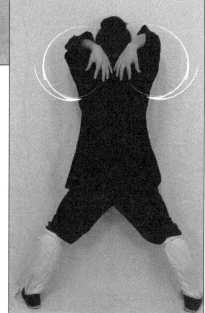

Figure 41a

Now, rotate your hands over and around your shoulders, under your armpits, and to your upper back. (Figures 42, 42a) Continue tapping down to your lower back. When you reach the level of your waist, make the sound "*Hai hei* 嗨嘿" (make this sound with your mouth closed, and feel as though the sound is coming from your kidneys) while imagining that you are sending the Qi to your kidneys. (Figure 42b)

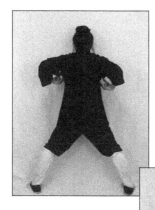

Figure 42

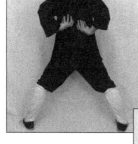

Figure 42a

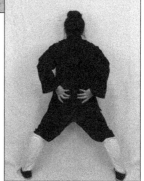

Figure 42b

Tap down your lower back and buttocks, down the outside of your upper legs, lower legs, and feet, crouching as you go. (Figures 43, 43a)

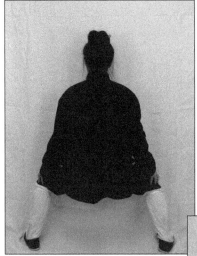

Figure 43

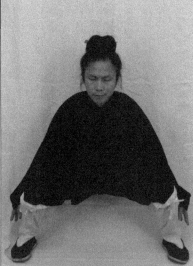

Figure 43a

Gathering the Earthly Qi: From a crouching position, sweep your hands around to the inside of your feet, and imagine that you are gathering the earthly Qi with your fingertips. (Figure 44)

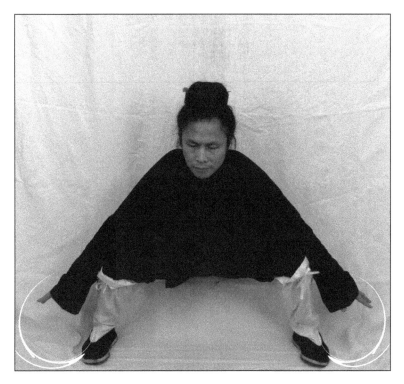

Figure 44

Tapping the Foot Yin Meridians: With strong fingers and a loose wrist, tap along your three Foot Yin Meridians. Starting from the inside of your feet, tap up through the inside of your lower legs and upper legs. Continue tapping along the midline of your abdomen, all the way up until you reach your chest. (Figures 45, 45a, 45b, 45c)

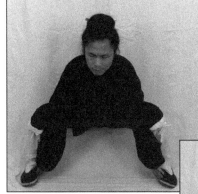

Figure 45

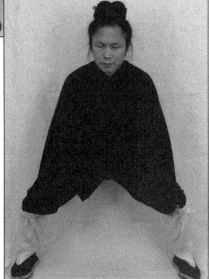

Figure 45a

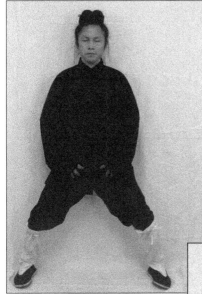

Figure 45b

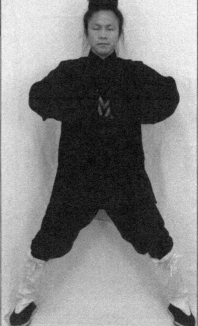

Figure 45c

Tapping the Belt Meridians: Take a deep breath. Turn your palms down, with fingertips pointing towards each other. (Figure 46) With the exhale, press your hands all the way down to the *DanTian* while sounding the mantra "*Heng* 哼" with your mouth closed. Feel as though the sound is coming from your *DanTian*. (Figure 46a)

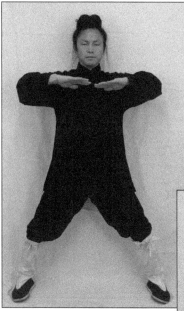

Figure 46

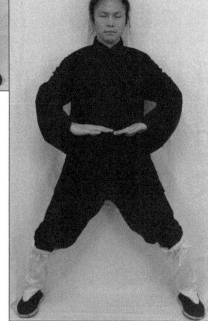

Figure 46a

Next, tap along the Belt Meridian from front to back and imagine sending the universal Qi into your body through your fingertips. (Figure 47) Make the sound *"Hai hei"* with a closed mouth as you tap your kidneys. (Figure 47a) Feel as though the sound is coming from your kidneys.

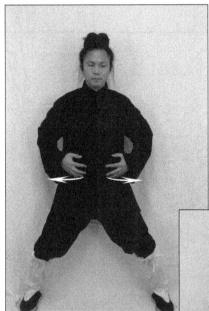

Figure 47

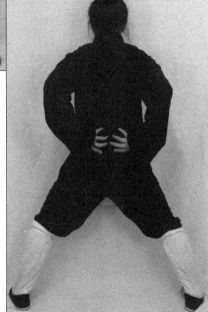

Figure 47a

Continue tapping along the Belt Meridian from back to front. Tap all around your *DanTian*, in the eight directions. (Figures 48, 48a, 48b)

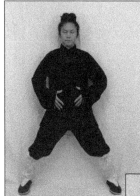

Figure 48

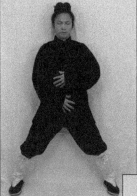

Figure 48a

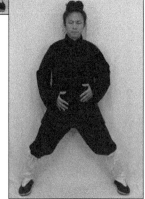

Figure 48b

End with your hands in front of the *DanTian*. (Figure 49)

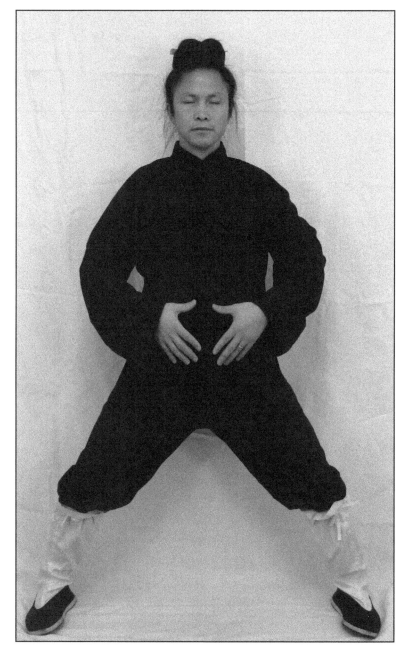

Figure 49

Function

This practice helps the smooth flow of Qi throughout the fifteen main meridians in your body, optimizing communication between and among your organs and the meridian system. Tapping these meridians will also awaken your hibernating dragons, thereby strengthening your inner fire, releasing areas of stagnation in your body, and regenerating your life energy.

5.5

YuLongPanXuan
玉龍盤旋

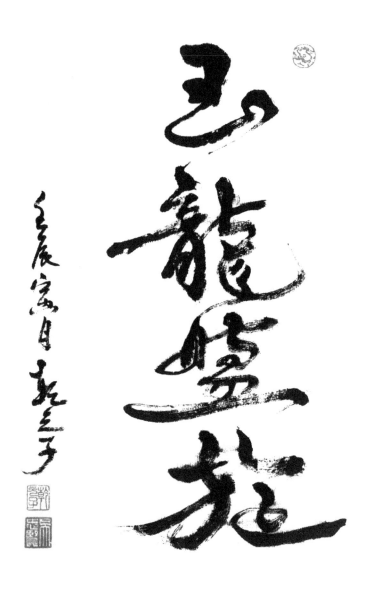

Jade Dragon Spins the Spiral

Movement

The sequence of this movement is almost exactly the same as the previous movement, *LongZhanYuYe*. There are two main differences between this portion of the Fire Dragon Meridian Qigong form and the previous one. First, during this section, we will not tap the meridians. Instead, we will go through the same loop guiding the Qi through the meridians. In order to guide the flow of Qi, you will not be touching your body. Instead, keep your hands about 3–5 inches away from the surface of your body and guide the Qi with the palm of your hand and your fingers. The second modification is your visualization. Instead of sending universal Qi into your meridians as you did previously, during the next section you will imagine the Qi current flowing through your meridians like a flying fire dragon.

The Rising Dragon: Slowly raise your arms so that your left arm is rounded in a full arc in front of your body at shoulder height and the right arm is rounded closer in towards your body at the level of your chest. Both palms should be facing your body. Next, spiral your hands, wrists, and arms with a spiraling motion that originates in your *DanTian*. Feel your entire body whorl like a rising dragon. (Figures 50, 50a)

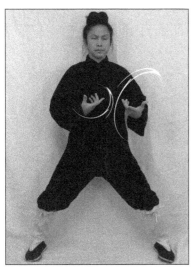 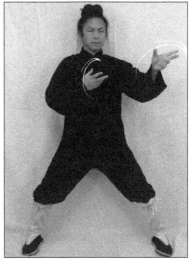

Figure 50   Figure 50a

Guiding the Qi through the Left Hand Yin Meridians: With an open palm and straight fingers, use your right hand to guide the Qi through the left-sided three Hand Yin Meridians. Starting from the center of your chest, guide the Qi through the inside of your left arm all the way to your palm and left fingertips. (Figures 51, 51a) Imagine the Qi is flowing through your meridians like a flying fire dragon as you move your right hand. When you finish, the left palm will be facing you and the right palm will face away from your body. (Figure 51b)

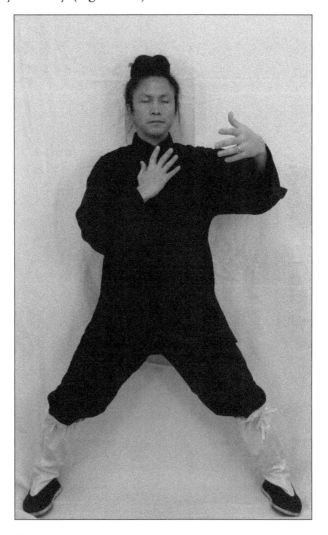

Figure 51

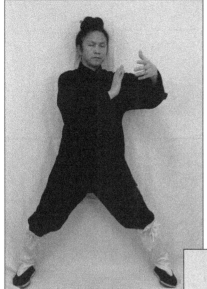

Figure 51a

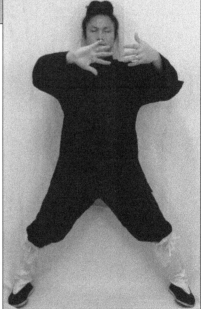

Figure 51b

Embracing the Pearl: Slowly turn over your left hand so that both palms face away from your body. With your fingers pointing towards each other, stretch your hands. Reach your pinky fingers towards heaven and extend your thumbs into the earth. (Figure 52)

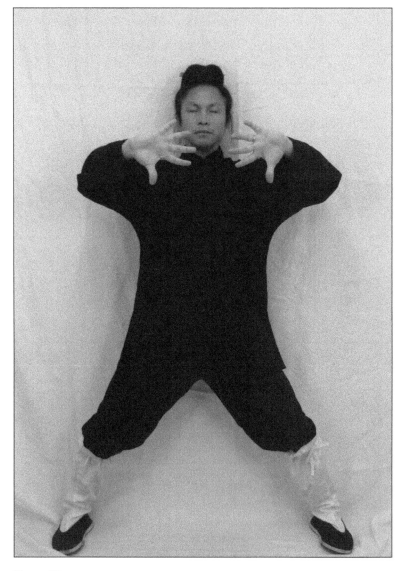

Figure 52

Feel the Qi connection between your hands. Continue to feel this connection as you pull your arms open to your side. With your palms facing away from you, open your chest. (Figure 53)

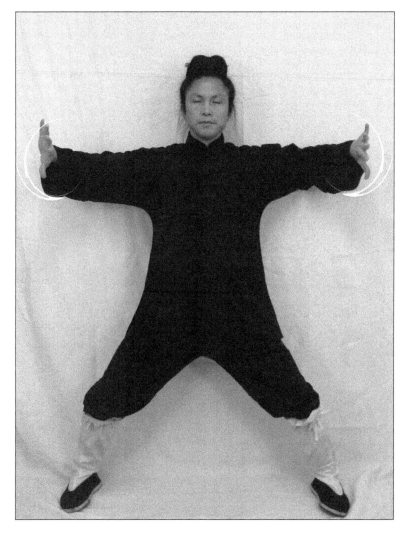

Figure 53

Next, rotating from your shoulders, turn your palms to face your body to embrace the Qi. Inhale and imagine you are holding a big ball of Qi. (Figure 54)

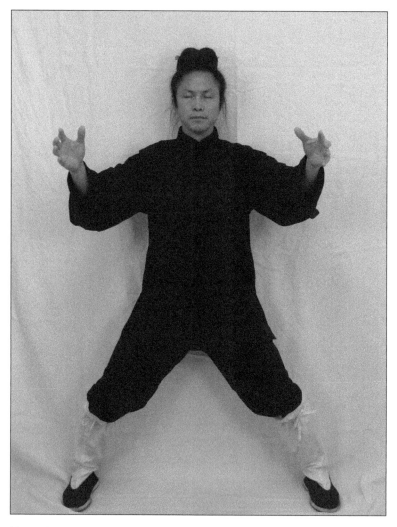

Figure 54

Exhale and circle your arms in front of you so that your fingertips almost touch. Do not touch your fingertips together. (Figure 55)

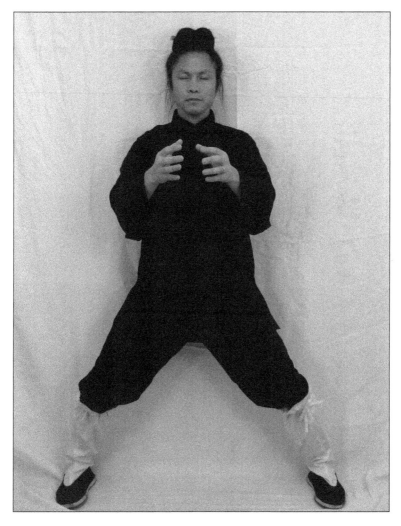

Figure 55

Inhale and gracefully open your arms again to embrace the Qi. (Figure 56)

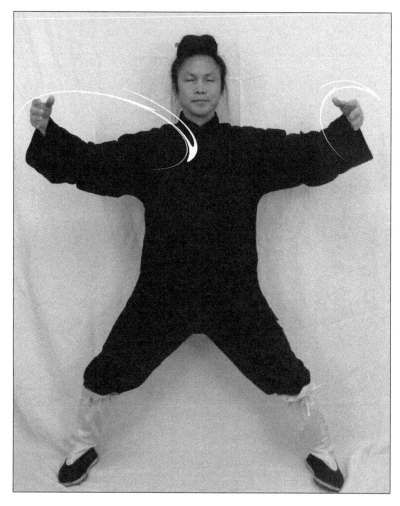

Figure 56

Turning Heaven and Earth: Open your left arm about 45 degrees from your body, with your left palm facing heaven. Feel your left hand connecting with heaven. At the same time, bend your right elbow and bring your right palm, facing earth, closer to your body at the level of your chest. Feel your right hand connecting with the earth. (Figure 57)

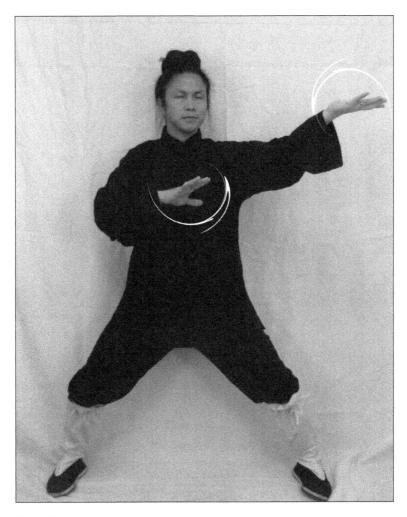

Figure 57

Spiral your hands one finger at a time so that your left palm now faces earth and your right palm faces heaven. (Figure 58)

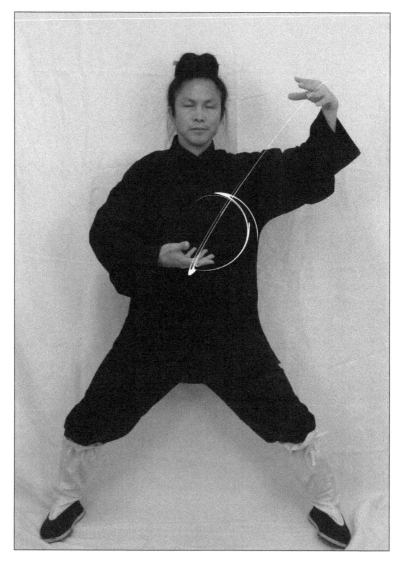

Figure 58

Bend your left arm, bringing your left hand to your chest, palm still facing earth. At the same time, rotate your right hand so that it now hovers, palm facing earth, directly over top of the left hand. (Figure 59)

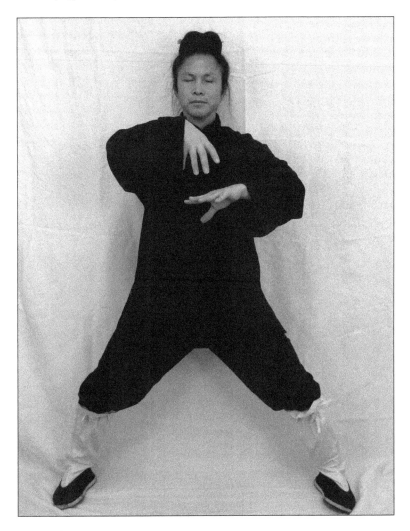

Figure 59

Guiding the Qi through the Left Hand Yang Meridians:
With your right hand, guide the Qi through your Left Hand
Yang Meridians. With your fingertips, guide the Qi to move from
your left fingers up along the outside of the left arm, across the
top of the left shoulder, up the side of your neck, and to the top
of your head. Imagine the Qi is flowing through your meridians
like a flying fire dragon as you go. (Figure 60) At the same time,
your left hand gradually moves downward until it reaches the
level of your Lower *DanTian*, with left palm facing earth. Imagine
pouring heavenly Qi into the Heavenly Gate on the top of your
head through your right hand. (Figure 60a)

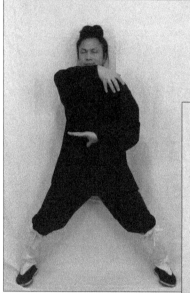

Figure 60

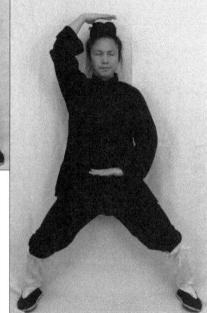

Figure 60a

The Rising Dragon: Rotate your right wrist, with the pinky finger moving around your ear and over the top of your shoulder, ending with the thumb by your ear. (Figure 61) Continue to move your right fingers away from you while extending your right arm. (Figure 61a)

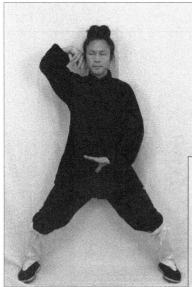

Figure 61

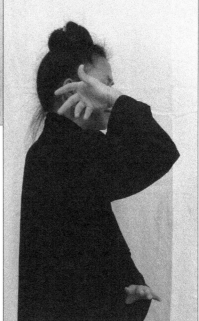

Figure 61a

As your right arm is extending from you at shoulder height, spiral your left hand upwards from your *DanTian* to the level of your chest. Rotate your hands, wrists, and arms with a spiraling motion that originates from your *DanTian*. Feel your entire body whorl like a rising dragon. (Figure 62)

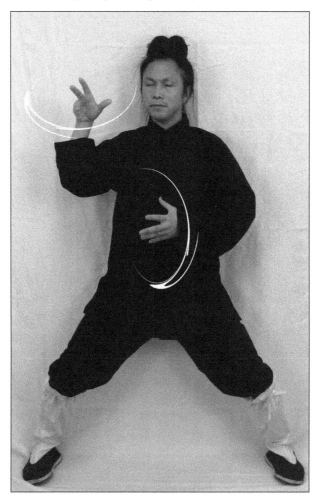

Figure 62

Guiding the Qi through the Right Hand Yin Meridians:
With an open palm and straight fingers, use your left hand to guide the Qi to flow through the right-sided three Hand Yin Meridians. Starting from the center of your chest, guide the Qi through the inside of your right arm all the way to your palm and right fingertips. Imagine the Qi is flowing through your meridians like a flying fire dragon as you go. When you finish, the right palm will be facing you and the left palm will face away from your body. (Figures 63, 63a, 63b)

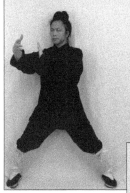

Figure 63

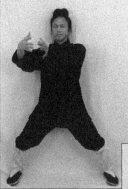

Figure 63a

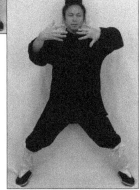

Figure 63b

Embracing the Pearl: Slowly turn over your right hand so that both palms face away from your body. With your fingers pointing towards each other, stretch your hands. Reach your pinky fingers towards heaven and extend your thumbs into the earth. (Figure 64)

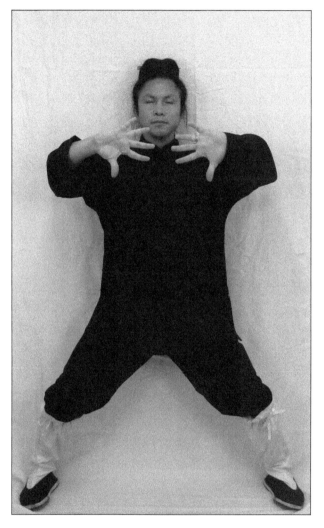

Figure 64

Feel the Qi connection between your hands. Continue to feel this connection as you pull your arms open to your side. With your palms facing away from you, open your chest. (Figure 65)

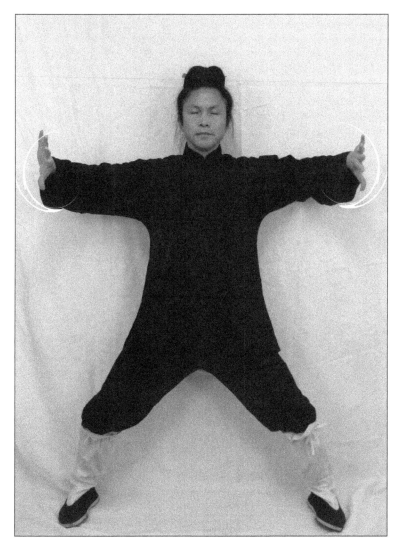

Figure 65

Next, rotating from your shoulders, turn your palms to face your body to embrace the Qi. Inhale and imagine you are holding a big ball of Qi. (Figure 66)

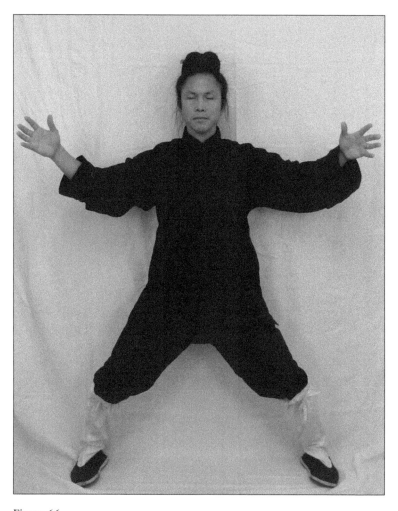

Figure 66

Exhale and circle your arms in front of you so that your fingertips almost touch. Do not touch your fingertips together. (Figure 67)

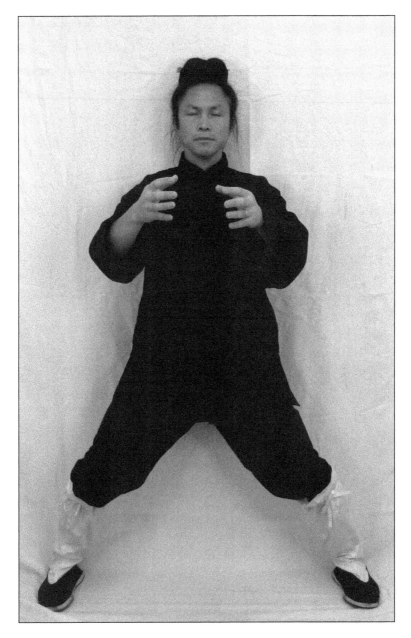

Figure 67

Inhale and gracefully open your arms to embrace the Qi again. (Figure 68)

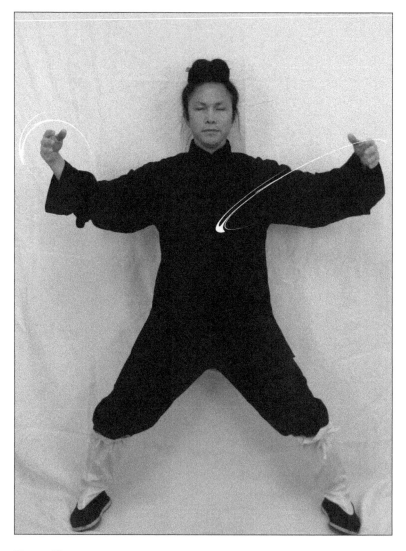

Figure 68

Turning Heaven and Earth: Open your right arm about 45 degrees from your body with your right palm facing heaven. Feel your right hand connecting with heaven. At the same time, bend your left elbow and bring your left palm, facing earth, closer to your body at the level of your chest. Feel your left hand connecting with the earth. (Figure 69)

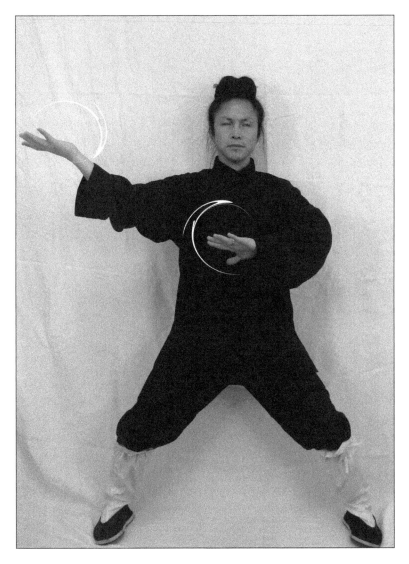

Figure 69

Spiral your hands one finger at a time so that your right palm now faces earth and your left palm faces heaven. (Figure 70)

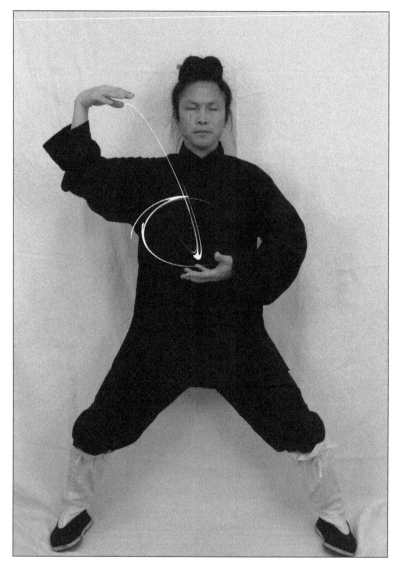

Figure 70

Bend your right arm, bringing your right hand to your chest, palm still facing earth. At the same time, rotate your left hand so that it now hovers, palm facing earth, directly over the top of the right hand. (Figure 71)

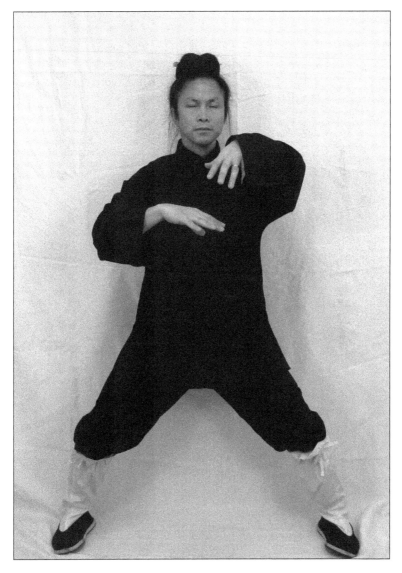

Figure 71

Guiding the Qi through the Right Hand Yang Meridians:
With your left fingers, guide the Qi through your Right Hand
Yang Meridians, moving from your right fingers up along the
outside of the right arm, across the top of the right shoulder, up
the side of your neck, and to the top of your head. Imagine that
the Qi is flowing through the meridians like a flying fire dragon
as you go. At the same time, your right hand gradually moves
downward until it reaches the level of your *DanTian*, with right
palm facing earth. (Figure 72) Imagine using your left hand to
pour heavenly Qi into the Heavenly Gate on the top of your
head. (Figure 72a)

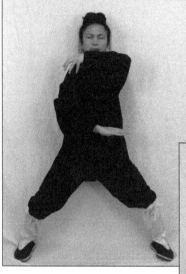

Figure 72

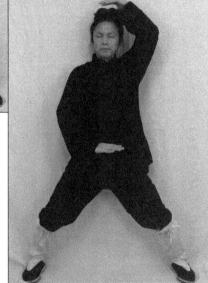

Figure 72a

Taking a Qi Shower: Rotate your left hand down along your left ear toward your left shoulder so that your left palm is cupped over your shoulder, close to your ear. (Figure 73) Swing your right arm up to reach the sky. (Figure 73a)

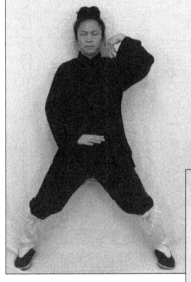

Figure 73

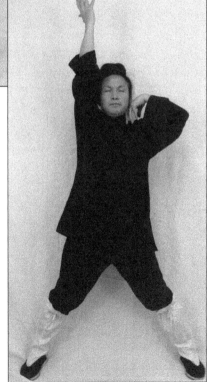

Figure 73a

Rotate your right fingers to grasp the heavenly Qi and bring your right hand, cupped, down to your right shoulder, close to your ear. Pour the Qi into your body through the top of your shoulder. Feel as though you are taking a Qi shower. (Figure 74) Next, squat down, as low as you can, while keeping your back straight. (Figure 74a)

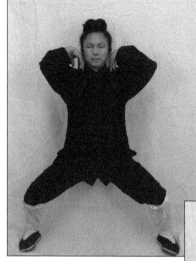

Figure 74

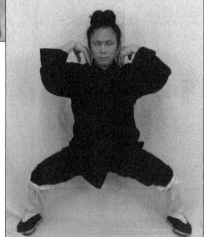

Figure 74a

In a squatting position, rotate your palms so that they face outward. Your hands are close to your ears and your fingers are pointing towards heaven. (Figure 75)

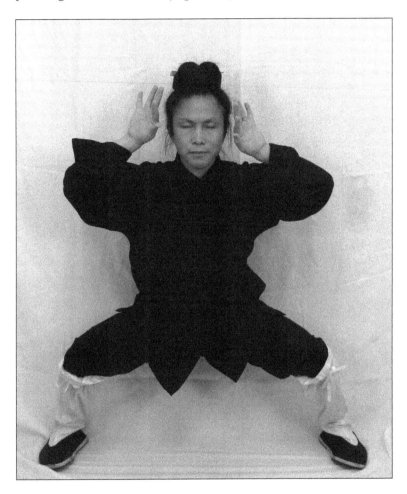

Figure 75

Straighten your legs and arms. Reach up with your fingertips and touch the heavens. Stretch and open one side of your body, then the other, alternating left and right. Imagine you are a dragon flying in the sky. (Figure 76)

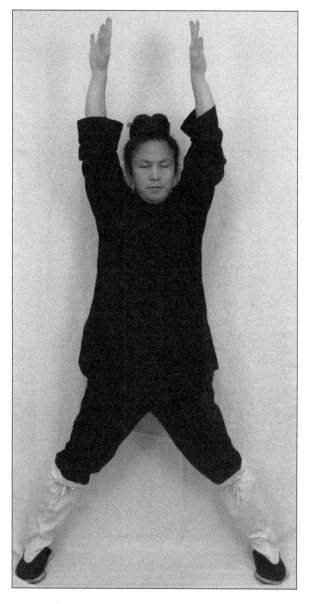

Figure 76

Rotate your hands to gather the heavenly Qi. (Figure 77) Lower your Qi-filled hands so they rest above the top of your head. Pour the Qi into your body through your Heavenly Gate. Feel as though you are taking a Qi shower. (Figure 77a)

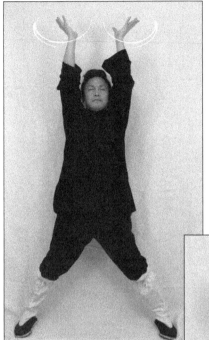

Figure 77

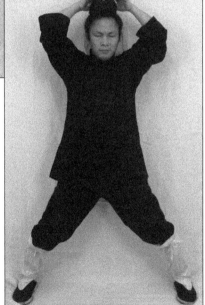

Figure 77a

Guiding the Qi through the Foot Yang Meridians: Next, bring your hands to the top of your head and begin guiding the Qi through your three Foot Yang Meridians. With an open palm and straight fingers, guide the Qi to move through the top of your head, the back of your head, your neck, and your upper back. (Figures 78, 78a)

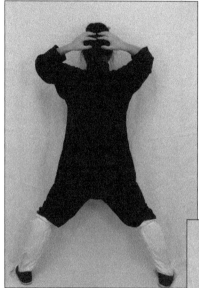

Figure 78

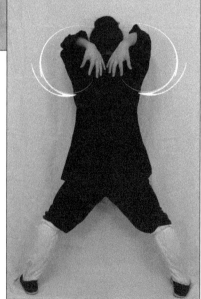

Figure 78a

Now, rotate your hands over and around your shoulders, under your armpits, and to your upper back. (Figure 79)

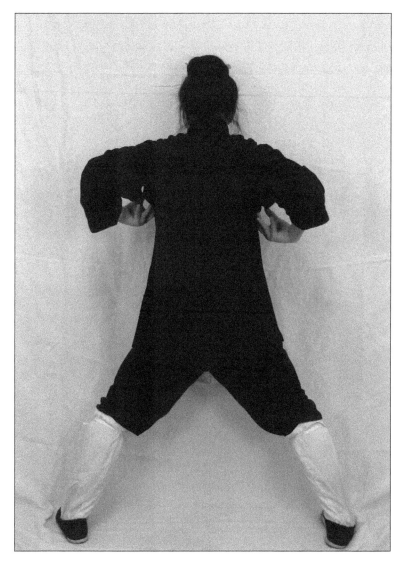

Figure 79

Continue guiding the Qi down your lower back. (Figure 80) When you reach the level of your waist, make the sound "*Hai hei*" (make this sound with your mouth closed, and feel as though the sound is coming from your kidneys) while imagining the Qi is swirling through your kidneys. (Figure 80a)

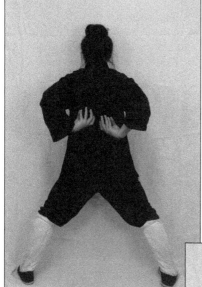

Figure 80

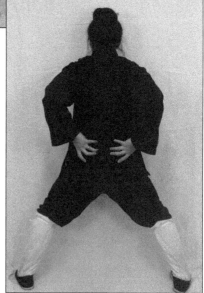

Figure 80a

Guide the Qi down your lower back and buttocks, down the outside of your upper legs, lower legs, and feet, crouching as you go. (Figure 81)

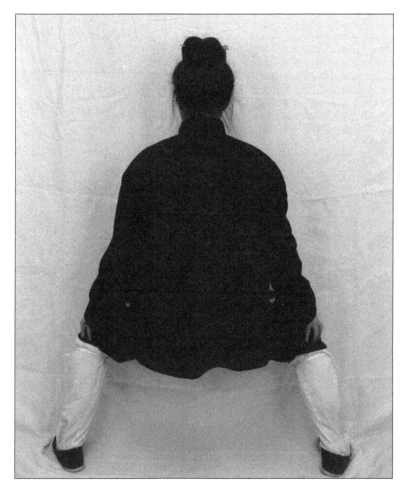

Figure 81

Gathering the Earthly Qi: From a crouching position, sweep your hands around to the inside of the feet, and imagine that you are gathering the earthly Qi with your fingertips. (Figure 82)

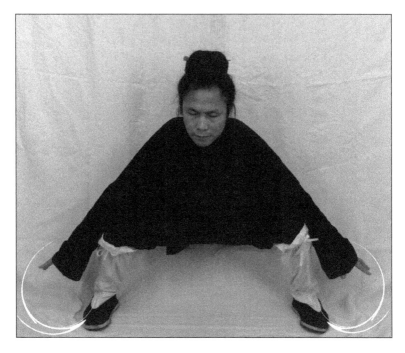

Figure 82

Guiding the Qi to move through the Foot Yin Meridians:
With your fingers, guide the Qi to move along your three Foot Yin Meridians. Starting from the inside of your feet, guide the Qi up through the inside of your lower legs and upper legs. (Figures 83, 83a)

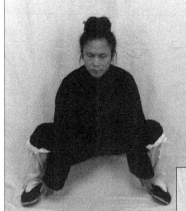

Figure 83

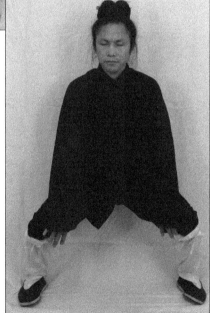

Figure 83a

Continue guiding the Qi along the midline of your abdomen, moving upwards until you reach your chest. (Figures 84, 84a)

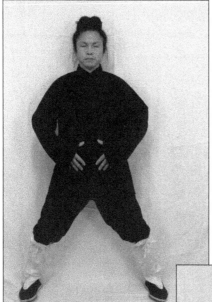

Figure 84

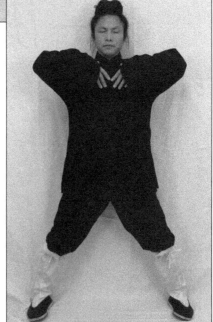

Figure 84a

Guiding the Qi through the Belt Meridians: Take a deep breath. Turn your palms down, with fingertips pointing towards each other. (Figure 85) With the exhale, press your hands all the way down to the *DanTian* while sounding the mantra *"Heng"* with your mouth closed. Feel as though the sound is coming from your *DanTian*. (Figure 85a)

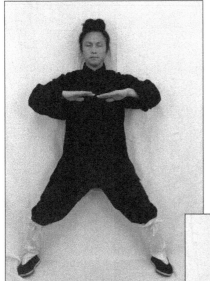

Figure 85

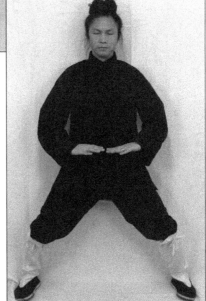

Figure 85a

Next, guide the Qi along the Belt Meridian from front to back and imagine the Qi is flowing through the meridian as you go. (Figure 86, 86a) Make the sound "*Hai hei*" with a closed mouth as you guide the Qi over your kidneys. (Figure 86b) Feel as though the sound is coming from your kidneys.

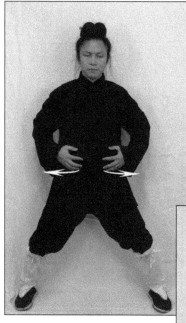

Figure 86

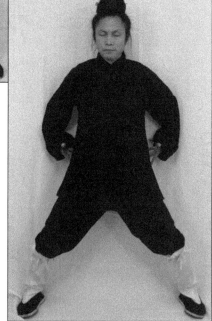

Figure 86a

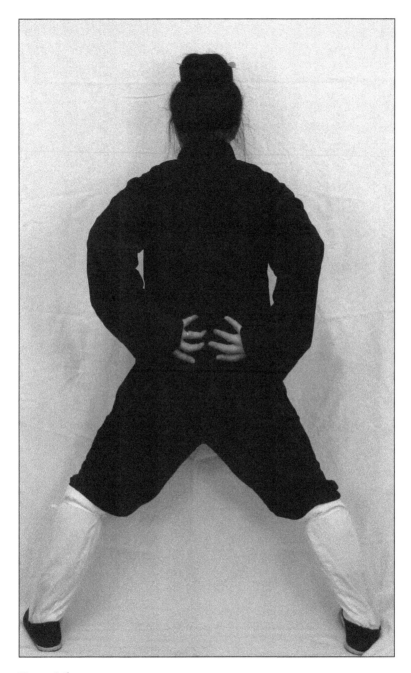

Figure 86b

Continue guiding the Qi along the Belt Meridian from back to front. Guide your Qi to move all around your *DanTian* in the eight directions. (Figures 87, 87a) End with your hands in front of the *DanTian*. (Figure 87b)

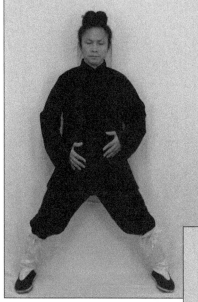

Figure 87

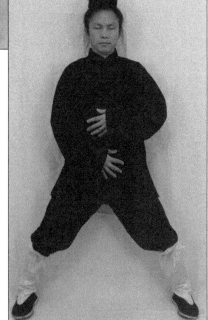

Figure 87a

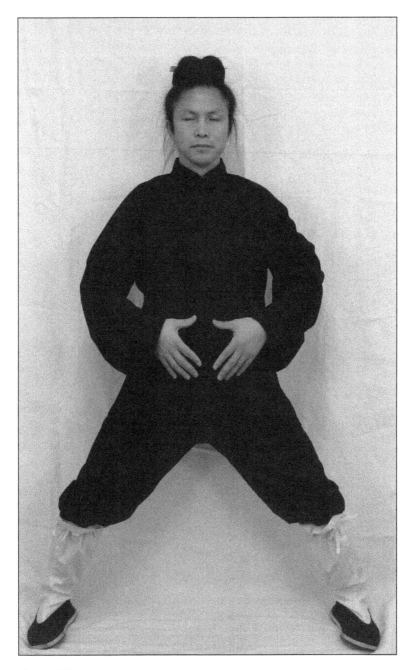

Figure 87b

Function

This practice intensifies the benefits of the tapping sequence and also strengthens your external and internal Qi. When we work with the fire dragon on this deeper level, we invite the opportunity for great inner transformation. With diligence in your daily practice, this movement will help you experience the process of refining your liquid that we discussed in Chapter 2. Working with the Qi in this more subtle way will increase your ability to do deep healing work, both on yourself and with others.

5.6

ShuangLongXiZhu
雙龍戲珠

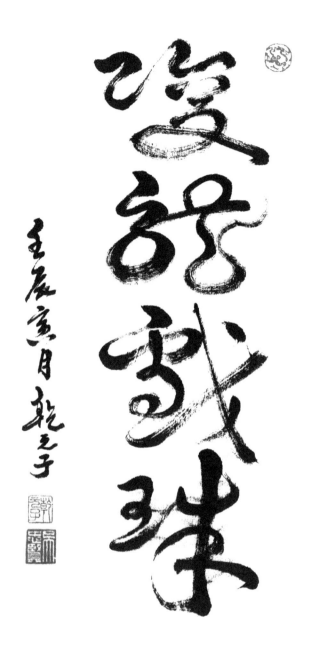

Double Dragons Play with the Pearl

Movement

Raise your right hand up through your midline, with your fingers pointing upward, and imagine your right fingertips reaching into the heavens. Lower your left hand along your midline, with your fingers pointing downward, and imagine your left fingertips extending into the center of the earth. Make sure your hands stay in the central line of your body. Your right palm is facing left and your left palm is facing right. (Figures 88, 88a)

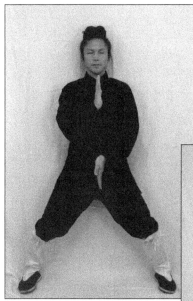

Figure 88

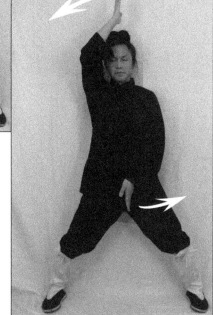

Figure 88a

Circle your arms open to the side and gather the universal Qi. Keep your palms facing each other. (Figure 89, 89a, 89b, 89c) Circle your right hand down to rest at the level of the Lower *DanTian*, with your right palm facing heaven. At the same time, circle your left hand up to rest at the level of your middle *DanTian* level, with your left palm facing earth. Imagine you are holding a ball of Qi between your hands. (Figure 89d)

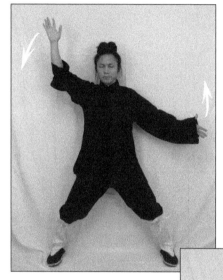

Figure 89

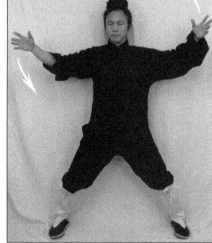

Figure 89a

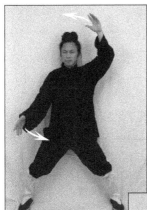

Figure 89b

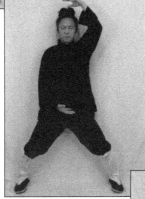

Figure 89c

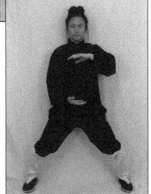

Figure 89d

Repeat this movement in the opposite direction:

Raise your left hand up through your midline, with your fingers pointing upward, and imagine your left fingertips reaching into the heavens. (Figure 90) Lower your right hand along your midline, with your fingers pointing downward, and imagine your right fingertips extending into the center of the earth. Make sure your hands stay in the central line of your body. Your left palm is facing right and your right palm is facing left. (Figure 90a)

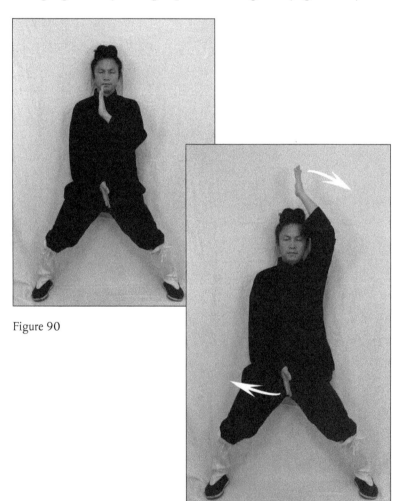

Figure 90

Figure 90a

Circle your arms open to the side and gather the universal Qi. Keep your palms facing each other. (Figures 91, 91a, 91b) Circle your left arm down to rest your hand at the level of the *DanTian*, with your left palm facing heaven. At the same time, circle your right arm up to rest your hand at the level of your middle *DanTian* level, with your right palm facing earth. Imagine you are holding a ball of Qi between your hands. (Figure 91c)

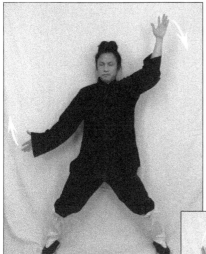

Figure 91

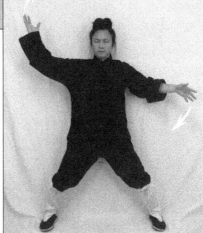

Figure 91a

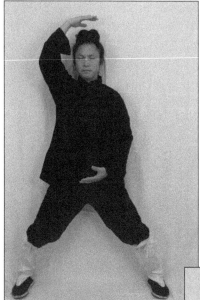

Figure 91b

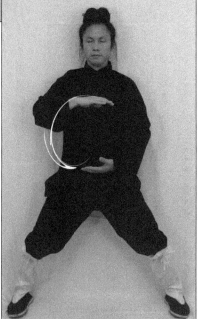

Figure 91c

Function

Practicing this movement will help balance your Yin Yang energy, and is especially beneficial for supporting the free flow of Qi, blood, and lymph through your body. This movement also strengthens your joints, organ systems, and *WeiQi* 外氣 (your external, protective Qi).

5.7

JinLongHuDing
金龍護鼎

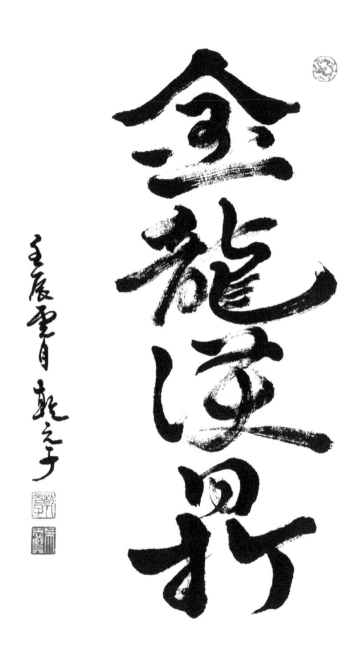

Golden Dragon Guards the Cauldron

Movement

Turn your right hand over and move it down to join the left hand at the level of your Lower *DanTian*. With both palms facing heaven, your fingertips will be pointing towards each other. (Figure 92)

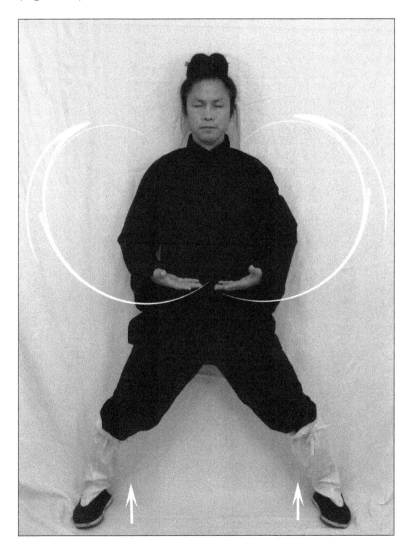

Figure 92

On your inhale, sweep your arms up until they are slightly higher than your head and, with an open chest, embracing heaven. At the same time, lift up onto your toes and turn your heels towards each other. (Figure 93)

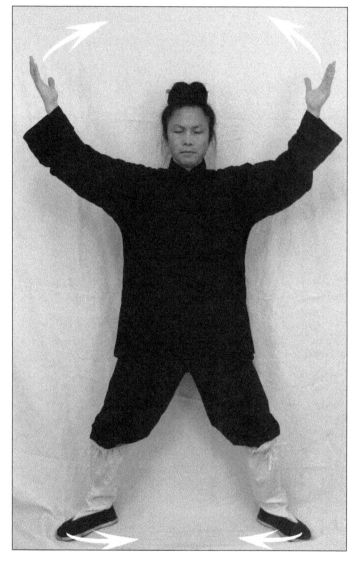

Figure 93

Lower your heels to the floor, turn your toes inwards towards each other, and circle your arms overhead so that your fingers point towards each other, palms facing earth. (Figure 94)

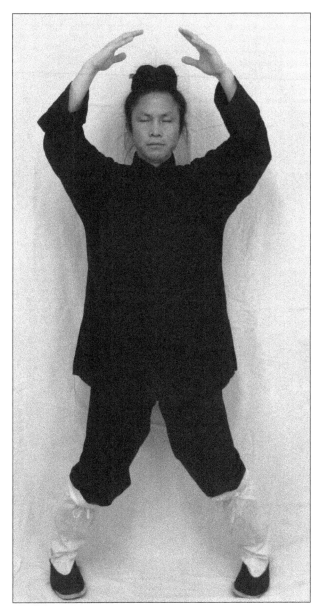

Figure 94

As you exhale, bring your hands straight down to your *Dan Tian.* (Figure 95)

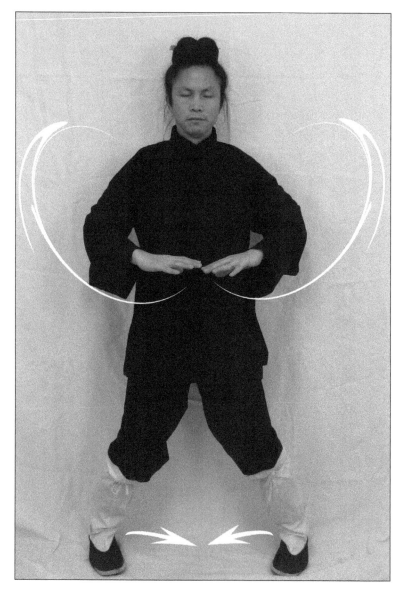

Figure 95

Repeat this sequence twice more so that you end with your feet together in a standing posture. (Figures 96, 96a, 96b, 96c, 96d, 96e)

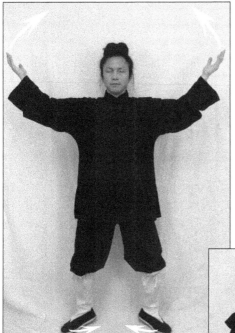

Figure 96

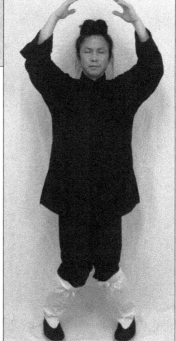

Figure 96a

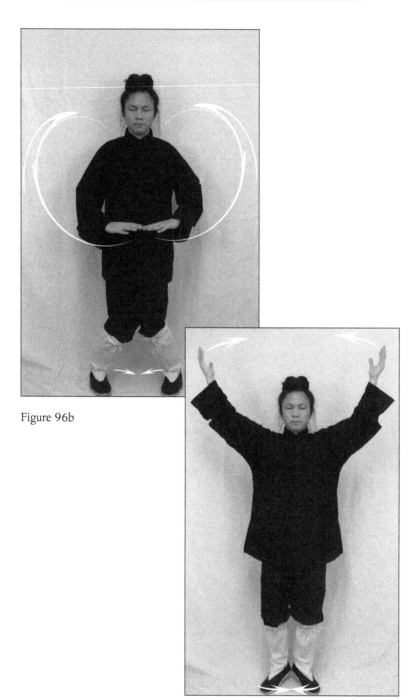

Figure 96b

Figure 96c

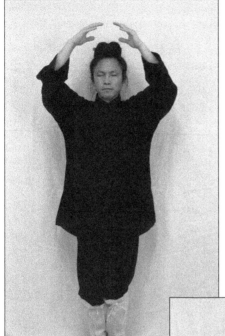

Figure 96d

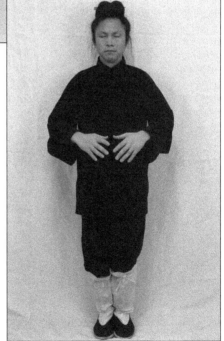

Figure 96e

Place your hands in *Taijiyin* 太極印, or Taiji Mudra. (Figure 97) In Chinese cultivation practices, we call the area in the curve between our thumb and index finger the "tiger mouth." To make the Taiji mudra, we place our tiger mouths together and rest our hands over our *DanTian*. Females will place their right hand inside the left, with the right palm touching the *DanTian*. Males will place their left hand inside the right, with the left palm touching the *DanTian*. The thumb of the outside hand touches the center of the palm of the inside hand. The thumb of the inside hand rests in the flesh between the thumb and index finger of the outside hand. Focus on your *DanTian*.

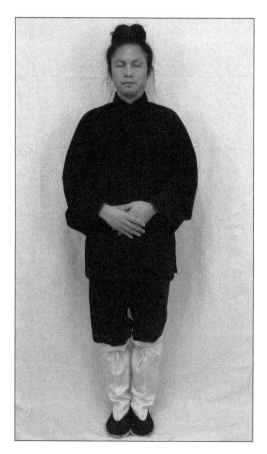

Figure 97

Great Transformation

FeiLongZaiTian
飛龍在天

Dragon is flying in the sky

YIJING

With the many changes in our lives this past year, karma steered us to the small coastal village Svarte, located on the southernmost tip of Sweden. The lulling and storming Baltic Sea, ancient burial mounds and stone circle, blossoming winter roses, and the constant flux of magical formations within the clouds inspired us to write this book together.

As we discussed in Chapter 2, the *Yijing* (*The Book of Change*) tells us to look to the clouds as guides when we seek the dragon. Yes, the clouds—the clouds follow the dragon. Where you see a cloud, you can be sure there is a dragon nearby. The dragon will always teach us something new when we observe the clouds in the sky. We would like to share with you our conversation with the dragon during our winter retreat:

The dragon, impulsively changing her shape, morphing from one formation into another as the clouds do their best to keep up, speaks in a slow and quiet voice, as though she were humming: "Life is fluid, just like my body—each moment, different and new. No one can live in a fixed way indefinitely."

While the moving clouds quickly dispersed in front of our eyes, the dragon questioned with her invisible body: "Where do my clouds go after they have vanished?"

"Where?" I meditate. "They are still in nature but in different configurations," I answered with a silent voice. "Is this the same reason the elders in my hometown use words like left, go back, or return when they talk about someone who has died?"

"Exactly. Life is just like my moving clouds," the dragon sang with her tranquil tones. "We are able to live in all places because we never desire to hold on to just one. We let ourselves transform as nature needs us to. Keep observing my clouds and you will find all the answers you seek."

This conversation deepened our insight into our inner cultivation practice and life itself. By observing the clouds, we have learned more about what is important about life and the purpose of our cultivation.

Many early mornings before dawn, we start our meditation with dark clouds cascading over the sea. We practice Gathering Sun Qi as the sun rises from the Baltic Sea like a flaming, floating pearl of the dragon. Gradually, the dark clouds transform into the dancing fire dragon. To us, this is the most exciting time for our cultivation practice, bringing us a sense of limitless joy and deep residing peace as the day begins.

Like a brilliant sunrise dancing over the sea, we hope your Fire Dragon Meridian Qigong practice will bring health, happiness, and peace in your daily life.

Master Zhongxian Wu
Dr. Karin Taylor Wu

LongYinGuan 龍吟館
(Singing Dragon Hermitage),
London, UK

February 2012, the arrival of RenChen 壬辰 *(Water Dragon)*

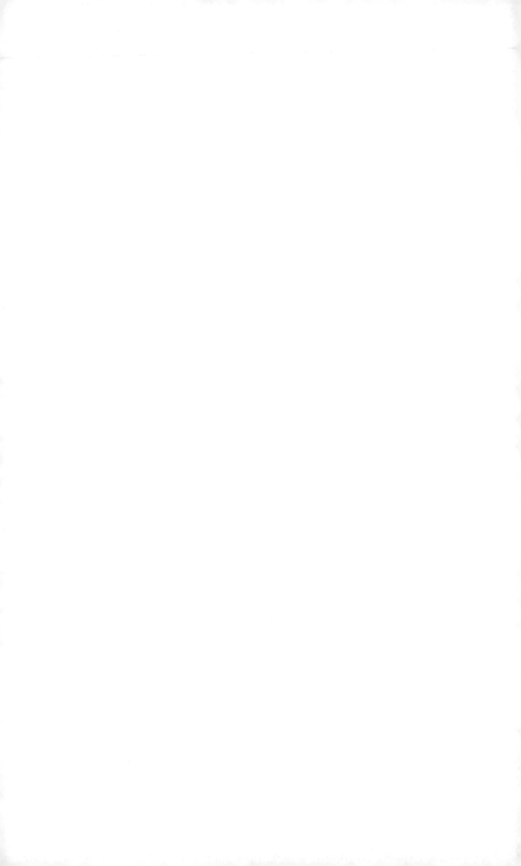

For Advanced Practitioners

Advanced Form—*JiBenGong* 基本功

Since I began teaching Qigong and martial arts in 1988, I have found that perhaps the most common question that arises for students is in regard to the advanced forms. "What is the most advanced form that I can learn? I want to: increase my energy level, improve my fighting skills, achieve Enlightenment (etc.)!" It is a natural inquiry for almost every Qigong, Taiji, other martial arts practitioner (including myself), or anyone else seeking a short cut—a way to accelerate the desired results—and one that can arise for people in all stages of their cultivation practice.

When I was very young, I searched for "The Advanced Form" and dreamed of transforming into the highest level—a most skillful martial artist or a superman. After all, in some of the fiction stories I read, the young hero would find the most secret master or receive the most secret transmission and would undergo an overnight metamorphosis. Luckily, it only took me a few years to find guidance from some illuminated masters who helped me realize what the advanced form truly is.

The most advanced practice is actually the *JiBenGong*—the basic, or fundamental, practices. *Ji* 基 originally refers to the foundation of a building. *Ben* 本 means the root of a tree. *Gong* 功,

as we discussed earlier, means to work hard in the correct way. The *JiBenGong* are the fundamental practices of any Qigong or martial arts form—the foundation on which the entire form rests that simultaneously contains the roots of the form's essence. After we learn how to practice a form, we must always go back to the root of the form—the primary elements that will help us move towards mastery, allowing our bodies to experience the form at its deepest levels and receive the most benefits from our practice.

For your review, please find the components that will, in time, prove to be the key that unlocks the transformative potential of the Fire Dragon Meridian Qigong form:

- Toes grab the earth
- Head upright
- Back straight
- Open *Tianmen* 天門 (Heavenly Gate)
- Seal *Dihu* 地戶 (Earthly Door)
- Build *QueQiao* 鵲橋 (Magpie Bridge)
- Keep your teeth and mouth closed
- *ShenGuangHuiShou* 神光回收 (Look within)
- Breathe with lungs and your skin
- Focus on your *DanTian* 丹田

Twelve Organ Meridian Charts

Once you master the physical details of form as described throughout this book, and can remember to maintain the *JiBenGong* throughout your entire practice, you will be ready for the next step—beginning to master the spirit of the form. This may take anywhere from six months to three years (or even longer), depending on your commitment to your daily practice.

Remember, *Gong* 功 tells us to work hard, in the correct way. You will have to pass through the stage where you practice to the point of feeling pain and exhaustion, with trembling body tissues and shaking thighs. You will be dripping with sweat from the tremendous internal heat generated by your physical exertion.

After you move through this stage, you will feel enlivened, surrounded, and refreshed by universal Qi. This indicates the beginning of new and transformed life energy. This may be the time for you to add the detailed visualization of the meridian systems of your body. Doing so will help you experience the movement of Qi throughout your body and the meridian systems, and may be of special interest to those of you who are Chinese medicine practitioners.

In this appendix, we have included the twelve organ meridian charts (with figures hand-drawn by Dr. Karin Taylor Wu and Chinese calligraphy by Master Zhongxian Wu). As the model for these charts, we chose a version based on the work of the eminent Chinese medicine doctor, *HuaShou* 滑壽, from 1341 CE. You may realize that these meridian charts are not as precise as the modern anatomically based meridian charts that are common today. In China, the traditional style of study stresses the importance of experiential learning over a mechanistic style of following a book. We added these charts to assist your visualization practice in the hope that you will discover the existence of the meridian systems of your body through your own direct experience.

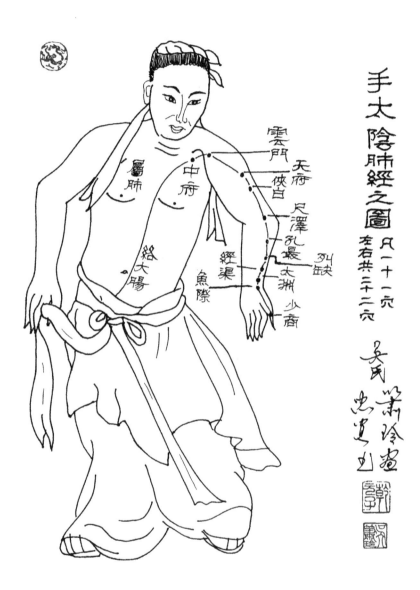

I. Hand Taiyin Lung Meridian

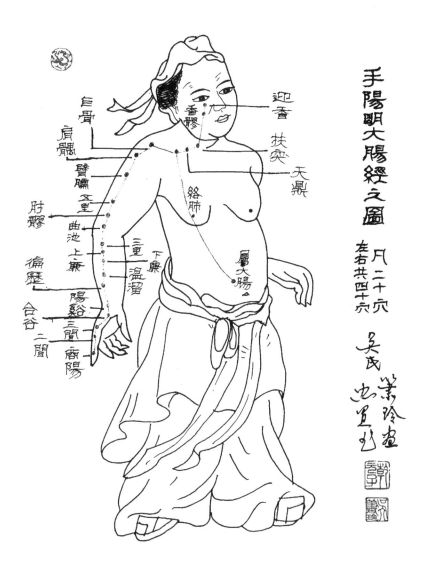

II. Hand Yangming Large Intestine Meridian

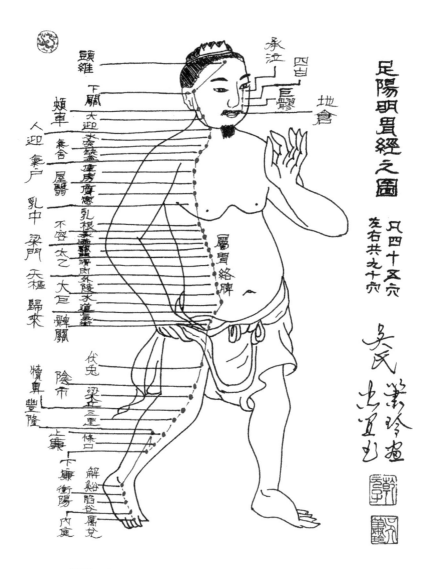

III. Foot Yangming Stomach Meridian

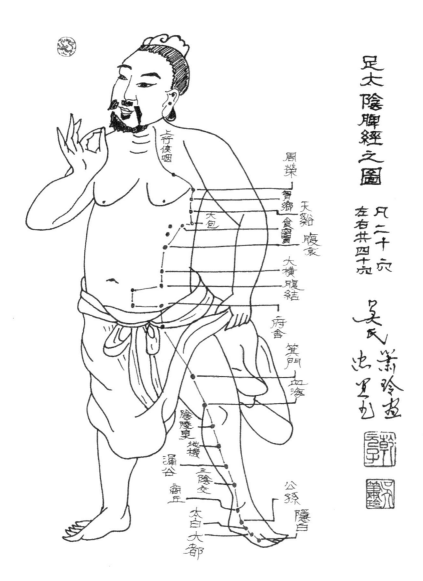

IV. Foot Taiyin Spleen Meridian

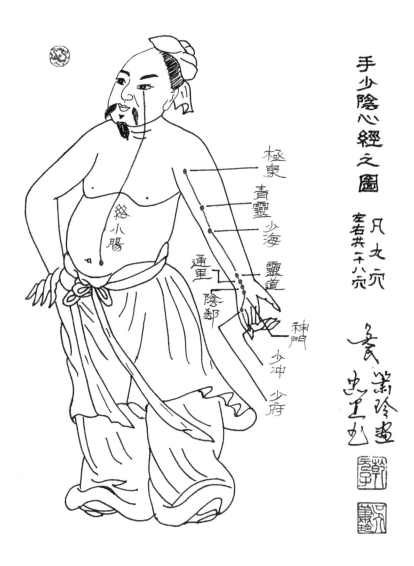

手少陰心經之圖　凡九穴　左右共十八穴

極泉
青靈
少海
靈道
通里
陰郤
神門
少衝　少府

絡小腸

V. Hand Shaoyin Heart Meridian

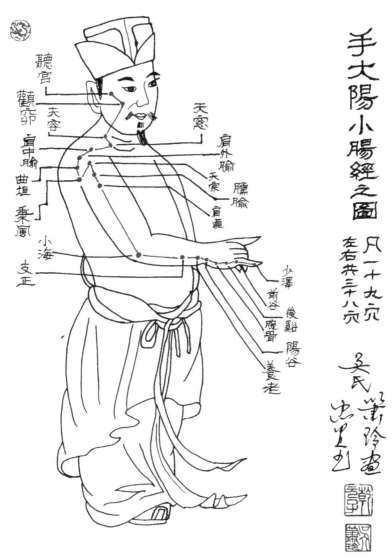

VI. Hand Taiyang Small Intestine Meridian

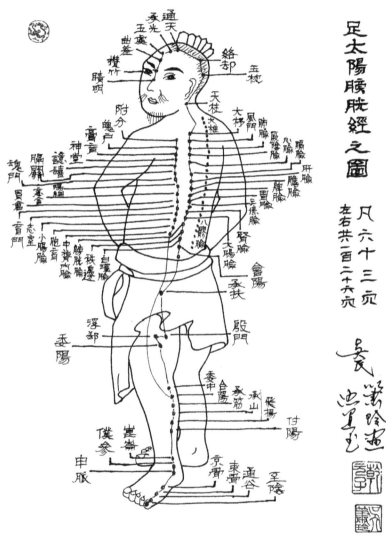

VII. Foot Taiyang Bladder Meridian

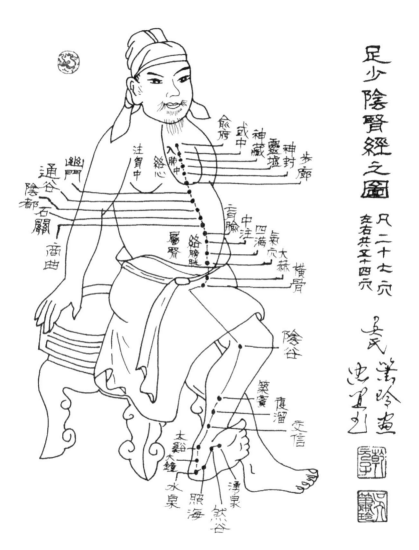

VIII. Foot Shaoyin Kidney Meridian

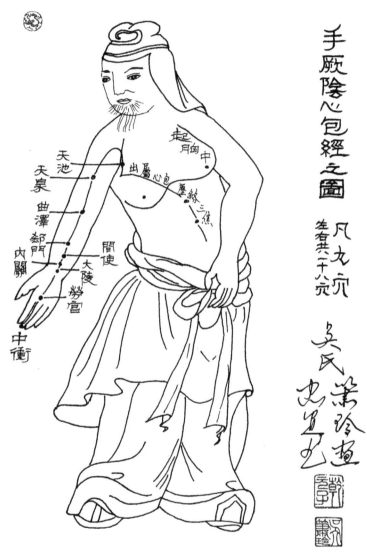

IX. Hand Jueyin Pericardium Meridian

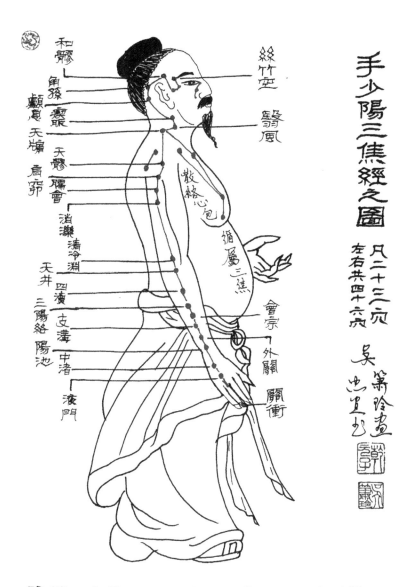

和髎
角孫
顱息 瘈脈
天牖 肩顒
天髎 臑會
消濼 清冷淵
天井 四瀆
三陽絡 支溝
陽池 中渚
液門

散絡心包
循屬三焦

絲竹空
翳風

會宗
外關
關衝

手少陽三焦經之圖
凡二十三穴
左右共四十六

吳忠望畫

X. Hand Shaoyang Triple Burner Meridian

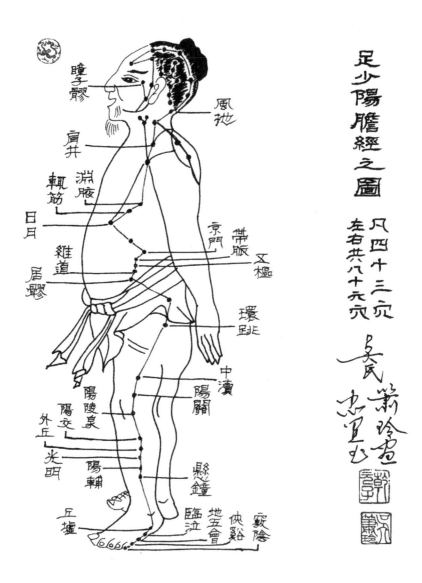

瞳子髎
風池
肩井
輒筋
淵腋
日月
京門
帶脈
維道
五樞
居髎
環跳
中瀆
陽關
陽陵泉
陽交
外丘
光明
陽輔
懸鐘
丘墟
臨泣
地五會
俠谿
竅陰

足少陽膽經之圖

凡四十三穴 左右共八十六穴

XI. Foot Shaoyang Gallbladder Meridian

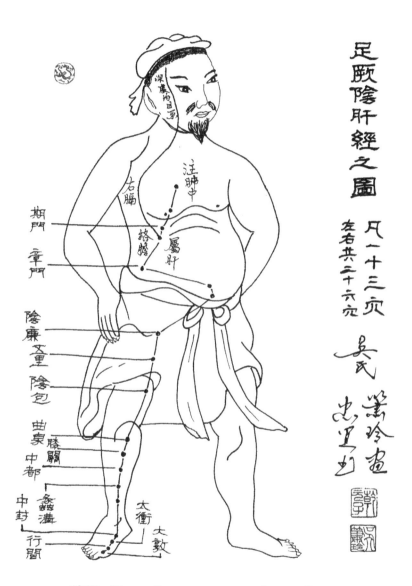

XII. Foot Jueyin Liver Meridian

Advanced Meridian Visualization Technique

Repeat "Dragon Battles on the Field" three times before moving to "Jade Dragon Spins the Spiral."

1. First time

    a. Tap the Hand Yin Meridians and visualize the image of the Lung Meridians.

    b. Tap the Hand Yang Meridians and visualize the image of the Large Intestine Meridians.

    c. Tap the Foot Yang Meridians and visualize the image of the Stomach Meridians.

    d. Tap the Foot Yin Meridians and visualize the image of the Spleen Meridians.

2. Second time

    a. Tap the Hand Yin Meridians and visualize the image of the Heart Meridians.

    b. Tap the Hand Yang Meridians and visualize the image of the Small Intestine Meridians.

    c. Tap the Foot Yang Meridians and visualize the image of the Bladder Meridians.

    d. Tap the Foot Yin Meridians and visualize the image of the Kidney Meridians.

3. Third time

    a. Tap the Hand Yin Meridians and visualize the image of the Pericardium Meridians.

    b. Tap the Hand Yang Meridians and visualize the image of the Triple Burner Meridians.

c. Tap the Foot Yang Meridians and visualize the image of the Gallbladder Meridians.

d. Tap the Foot Yin Meridians and visualize the image of the Liver Meridians.

Next, repeat "Jade Dragon Spins the Spiral" three times, using the same visualization technique listed above. Remember, for this movement you will not be tapping the meridians; rather, you will be guiding the Qi to move through the meridians.

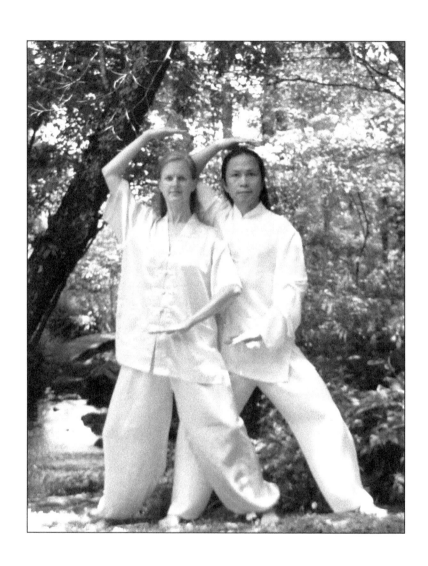

About the Authors

Master Zhongxian Wu was born on China's eastern shore in the city of Wenling in Zhejiang Province, where the sun's rays first touch the Chinese mainland. He began practicing Qigong and Taiji at an early age. Inspired by the immediate strengthening of this practice, Master Wu committed himself to the life-long pursuit of the ancient arts of internal cultivation.

In 2001, Master Wu left his job as an aerospace engineer in Xi'an, China, to teach in the United States. For four years he served as Senior Instructor and Resident Expert of Qigong and Taiji in the Classical Chinese Medicine School of the National College of Natural Medicine (NCNM) in Portland, Oregon. In addition to his work at NCNM, Master Wu was a sub-investigator in a 2003 Qigong research program sponsored by the National Institute of Health (NIH).

Master Wu has published nine books (five of which were written and published in China), and numerous articles on the philosophical and historical foundations of China's ancient life sciences, including the first book in English on Chinese Shamanic Qigong, *Vital Breath of the Dao: Chinese Shamanic Tiger Qigong—Laohu Gong*.

Since he began teaching in 1988, Master Wu has instructed thousands of Qigong students, both eastern and western. Master

Wu is committed to bringing the authentic teachings of Chinese ancient wisdom traditions such as Qigong, Taiji, martial arts, calligraphy, Chinese astrology, and Yijing science to his students. He synthesizes wisdom and experience for beginning and advanced practitioners, as well as for patients seeking healing, in his unique and professionally designed courses and workshops. He also offers a long-term Qigong training program which provides a strong foundation for the study of shamanic Qigong, internal alchemy, Taiji, and Qi-healing skills (including classical Chinese energy techniques, Chinese calligraphy, medical Qigong, and martial arts applications). Please visit www.masterwu.net for further details about his teachings.

Dr. Karin Taylor Wu is a medically trained naturopathic physician, who graduated from one of the seven federally accredited medical schools in North America that train primary care physicians in complementary and alternative medicine.

After obtaining a bachelor's degree in biology from the University of Colorado, she traveled widely, exploring the nature of the human mind and traditional medicines from cultures around the globe. She began in-depth studies of the Five Element System, a Daoist, nature-based approach to Chinese medicine, in 2004. This elegant system continues to hold her framework for understanding the cycles of life and living, thereby bridging eastern and western understandings of health and healing in individuals, communities, and in the earth herself.

With the strengths of modern science and ancient wisdom to draw on, Dr. Taylor Wu combines recommendations for breath work, nutrition, movement, and sleep habits with natural therapies (including herbal medicines, nutritional supplements, homeopathy, hydrotherapy, and cranial therapy) into individualized health plans targeted towards revitalizing the body, balancing the mind, and uplifting the spirit.

Dr. Taylor Wu currently serves as medical director of Blue Willow World Healing Center, which offers a variety of services aimed at restoring optimal health and inspiring people to enrich the quality of their lives by making the sustainable choices that create balance and harmony in themselves and in the world at large.

Fire Dragon Meridian Qigong
Essential NeiGong for Health
and Spiritual Transformation
Master Zhongxian Wu
ISBN: 978 1 84819 111 2
DVD video
£25.00/US$39.95

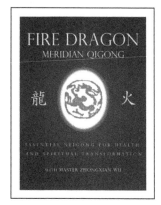

Fire Dragon Meridian Qigong is a remarkably powerful practice developed to revitalize our health and deepen our spiritual connection to the Dao. Lineage holder, Master Zhongxian Wu provides detailed instruction in this powerful form from the EmeiZhenGong school. It is an ancient Wu (Chinese shamanic) style Qigong form. The Wu tradition is the source of all classical Chinese culture, including Confucianism, Daoism, Chinese medicine, and the martial arts.

For thousands of years, the dragon has been an auspicious symbol of transformation throughout China. Fire Dragon Meridian Qigong works directly with the body's meridian systems, transforming areas of Qi stagnation into a free flowing state, thereby strengthening the body, balancing the mind, and reuniting us with our original nature. It is a Qigong form that is specifically recommended for people seeking healing from cancer and other serious chronic health conditions.

This DVD includes detailed instruction of the form, including Master Wu's interpretation of the meaning of each movement from a NeiGong (internal alchemy) perspective, as well as demonstration of the entire form.